RINNAVATI✿N

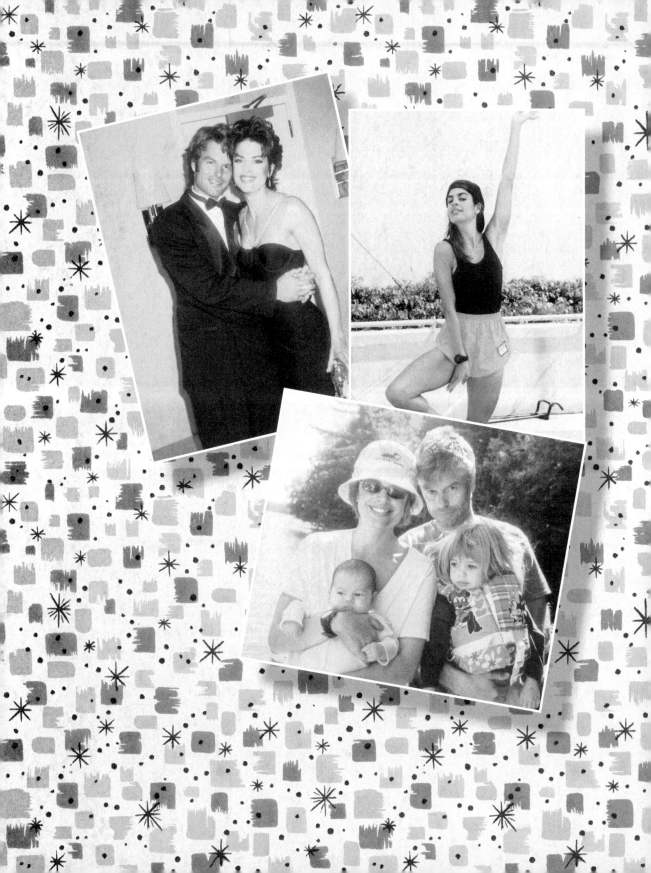

RINNAVATIN

GETTING YOUR BEST LIFE EVER

LISA RINNA

SSE

SIMON SPOTLIGHT ENTERTAINMENT

New York London Toronto Sydney

NOTE TO READERS

This publication contains the opinions and ideas of its author. It is intended to provide help-ful and informative material on the subjects addressed in the publication. It is sold with the understanding that the author and publisher are not engaged in rendering medical, health, fitness, or any other kind of personal professional services in the book. The reader should consult his or her medical, health, or other competent professional before adopting any of the suggestions in this book or drawing inferences from it.

In addition, this book sometimes recommends particular products for your reference. Unless otherwise indicated in the text, the author is not affiliated in any way with such products or the companies that produce them. In all instances, bear in mind that there are products other than those recommended here that you may find useful.

The author and publisher specifically disclaim all responsibility for any liability, loss, or risk, personal or otherwise, which is incurred as a consequence, directly or indirectly, of the use and application of any of the contents of this book.

SIMON SPOTLIGHT ENTERTAINMENT
A Division of Simon & Schuster, Inc.
1230 Avenue of the Americas
New York, NY 10020

First Simon Spotlight Entertainment hardcover edition May 2009

SIMON SPOTLIGHT ENTERTAINMENT and colophon are trademarks of Simon & Schuster, Inc.

For information about special discounts for bulk purchases, please contact Simon & Schuster Special Sales at 1-866-506-1949 or business@ simonandschuster.com

The Simon & Schuster Speakers Bureau can bring authors to your live event. For more information or to book an event contact the Simon & Schuster Speakers Bureau at 1-866-248-3049 or visit our website at www.simonspeakers.com.

Designed by Dana Sloan

Manufactured in the United States of America

10   9   8   7   6   5   4   3   2   1

Library of Congress Cataloging-in-Publication Data
Rinna, Lisa.
    Rinnavation : getting your best life ever / Lisa Rinna.
        p. cm.
    1. Rinna, Lisa. 2. Women—Conduct of life. 3. Beauty, Personal.
4. Spiritual life. I. Title.
    BJ1547.5.R56A3 2009
    155.3'33—dc22
                                                            2009005590

ISBN-13: 978-1-4169-4863-6
ISBN-10:   1-4169-4863-5

To my angels, Delilah and Amelia.

This is for you! Thank you for showing me the way.

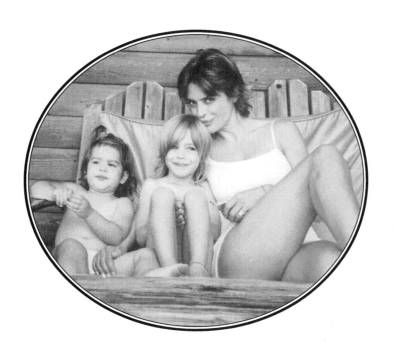

CONTENTS

FOREWORD

BY HARRY HAMLIN

The summer of 1992 was momentous for me. My mother died in early July, my wife ran off with a pop singer in mid-July, and I met Lisa Deanne Rinna in late July. It was not the kind of July I was used to.

I remember clearly the emotional impact of each of those events. The first two caused fairly predictable reactions—I grieved for my mother and was saddened and enraged by my wife's behavior. But sooner or later all our parents pass on and, sooner or later, if you marry a certain kind of person, they're going to run off. It was meeting Lisa that was most astonishing.

We met on a balmy night at one of Wolfgang Puck's smaller trattorias, high up in the hills of Bel Air. I was commiserating with a friend over a glass of pinot noir about the demise of my yearlong marriage, when a pretty brunette in jeans and a T-shirt strolled up to our table and handed a set of keys to my friend. I stood; I heard my friend introduce her as "Lisa Renneau," the night sales-girl at his eyeglass store, which was next door to the restaurant. She had closed up and was returning the keys.

I was vaguely annoyed that our conversation—a lengthy diatribe by me about the horrible month I was having—had been interrupted, and I just wanted her to go away so I could get back to "poor me." But as I shook her hand, I looked into her eyes and saw something that took my breath away. It was a kind of openness or willingness unobscured by any social mask or preening—an authenticity rare in the Hollywood ether. Her eyes said, "Here I am; what you see is what you get."

Now, at that moment the last thing on my mind was romance and, given the fact that I was an emotional wreck, the thought of having any real feelings for another woman was out of the question; but I was smitten and I couldn't help myself. I asked the night salesgirl with the exotic French name to join us.

She sat down and began to tell us about her experience seeing Cirque du Soleil, the new traveling acrobatic extravaganza from Canada that was the talk of the town. She described in detail, practically squealing from excitement, the various acts, and kept going on about how sexy it all was. Between that first look, her exotic French name, and her obsession with how sexy the circus was, I was hooked.

Later that night, in the parking lot of the restaurant, I told my friend that I had found Lisa enchanting and that I was surprised, given my current emotional state, that I could have any feelings at all for another woman. I told him that if I were a single man, I would like to see her again.

And see her again I did. A few weeks later, after I had filed for divorce, I called her up on a weeknight and asked if she would join me for dinner in an hour at my favorite Italian joint in Brentwood. I knew it was a long shot. Most girls were following the dating "advice" of other women (that would later be set forth in a book called *The Rules*), and were turning down any invitation from a man unless the date was at least three days away. But Lisa was "game," and one hour later she showed up in a T-shirt and jeans at Toscana for our first date. I asked about her French heritage and was informed that she was of Italian descent, that her name was Rinna, not Renneau, and that she did not hail from Saint Tropez but from a little-known small town in Oregon. I was only a little disappointed by that and remained optimistic, but still the date didn't go as well as I had hoped. Despite the fact that our waiter kept telling us in a thick Italian accent that we were destined to be together, our conversation was stilted. Then, after dinner in the parking lot as we said goodbye, I went in for the obligatory first date kiss, and it was a disaster—the kiss of death . . . nothing . . . *nada . . . niente.* I was definitely disappointed to say the least, and went home thinking that I would never find romance again.

Six months later, with another divorce behind me, I was once again a single man and I couldn't get Lisa out of my mind. By then, things had changed pretty radically in Lisa's life. No longer was she the night salesgirl at an eyeglass store; she had landed a plum role on the daytime soap *Days of Our Lives*. I'd forgotten about the rotten kiss, and it was the look, that first look, that I kept coming back to. I became obsessed. I called her every day trying to get some positive feedback, some hint that there might be a crack in the door. What was it about that look?

I called her up over the holidays and invited her to join me and my son on a ski trip in Colorado. This time she was not "game," and rightly so. What was I thinking? What, she's going to drop everything and fly to Colorado on the spur of the moment to hang out with a guy she doesn't know and his thirteen-year-old son?

I think that my respect for her went through the roof the more she rebuffed my advances; but clearly, as history shows, she eventually relented and we came together and have stayed together for sixteen years.

So what is it about little Lisa Rinna from Medford, Oregon, that put such a spell on me? I've gone back and thought about that first "look," and I've watched her for sixteen years and I think I know what it is. She's "game." The *Oxford English Dictionary* has this to say about Lisa's variety of the word "game": *Game* / a. 1. Like a gamecock: Full of fight: spirited, plucky. 2. Having the necessary will for, to do: ready and willing.

Cockfighting aside, she certainly is spirited, plucky, and full of fight, and that is what keeps me glued to her proverbial screen every single day. Lisa is totally willing to put herself out there, and she is totally committed to getting to the bottom of anything she decides to explore. She is absolutely committed once she decides to focus on something. Here's an example: Not long after we started seeing each other in earnest, we went to Hawaii for a three-day vacation. I've been an avid scuba diver since I was a teenager, and I asked if she wanted to try it. After a three-hour course in the hotel swimming pool, the instructor took us out on a shore dive to fifty feet. Lisa seemed to be doing fine and seemed to be enjoying herself. A lot of people get freaked out on their first dive to fifty feet. Suddenly, the instructor plucked an octopus from a crevice in some coral and put the darned thing over his face. It covered his mask and the tentacles wrapped around his neck! Even I, an old salty diver, was creeped out. He took the creature off his face and handed it to Lisa. I thought she would be having a cow about then, but no—she took the octopus and held it up to her face mask and that critter wrapped its two-foot-long tentacles around her head and neck in a split second.

Now just imagine . . . you've never dived underwater with a tank before, you're with a man you hardly know and a scuba instructor you've known for four hours, and you're at the bottom of the ocean with an octopus wrapped around your head. Anyone else would have drowned in their own vomit, but I could see Lisa smiling as we looked on. Now that's what I call "game"! Thus began a parade of "game" moments that have kept me in awe of her for sixteen years; from convincing Hugh Hefner that he needed to do a nude pictorial of a pregnant woman in her third trimester, to suiting up and conquering *Dancing with the Stars,* to many more moments in between.

Now Lisa's embarking on a new career as an inspirational author, speaker, and exercise guru. And why not? Because she is "game," Lisa has explored practically every exercise regime, diet plan, and spiritual path to self-evolution known to man. Since I've known her, she's studied everything from the Course in Miracles to Eckhart Tolle to Kaballah, and much more. She's mastered Tae Bo, yoga, pole dancing, and ballroom dancing, while keeping up a steady routine of working out in the gym, spinning, and aerobics. That makes me a lucky guy for sure. Make no mistake, we have worked hard on our relationship and that's what it takes to create a good marriage;

but it requires willingness from both people to make that work pay off. And that's what I saw in Lisa Rinna on that first balmy night in July of '92. I saw willingness. Now I call it "game," because even though a marriage requires work, it also has to be fun. And so we work at it, and we play at it, and still, little Lisa Rinna from Medford, Oregon, never ceases to surprise me. My guess is, as you read on, she'll surprise you too!

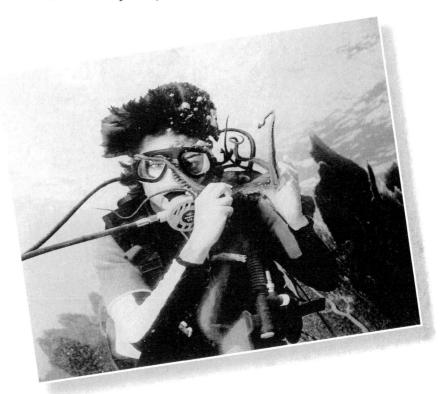

INTRODUCTION

I stood in my bedroom, naked, and looking in the mirror. It was not a pretty sight. I was thirty-eight years old, and had given birth to my second daughter the previous year. Despite a bout of soul-crushing postpartum depression (my second), I had managed to lose the thirty pounds I had gained, and my body was almost back to its pre-baby shape. But after breast-feeding two babies, my breasts hung from my chest like two pathetic, deflated balloons, and I felt about as sexual as a coat rack.

I hated looking in the mirror (not a healthy trait in anyone, let alone an actress). I felt unattractive, dried up, dead. My sex life with my husband was practically non-existent, but after ten years together and two kids, whose wasn't? That was what I told myself. I blamed it on our busy schedules, or the lingering effects of postpartum depression, but deep down I knew I was fooling myself. It was me—plain and simple. I didn't feel good about myself, and I transferred these feelings to my family, my marriage, my sex life, and my career (or in those days, the lack of one). I had been let go from my second stint on the soap opera *Days of Our Lives* the year before, after a two-year run on *Melrose Place*. To say I was in a rut was an understatement. I had set up camp there.

What had happened to me? I had what most people would kill for—a fabulous husband and soul mate, two exquisite daughters, a home in Beverly Hills, the career I had always dreamed of (current dry spell notwithstanding), and I was in good physical shape. I wondered if there was something in my genes that prevented me from appreciating what I had. Truth be told, despite my sunny exterior, I had never been a "happy" person. Throughout my twenties and thirties, I always carried a vague feeling of unease, the sense that *something* was missing. In the business I'm in, feeling insecure at times is part of the deal, but I'm pretty sure I would have felt the same way had I still been living anonymously, outside of Hollywood.

It's not as if I was a stranger to obstacles. Growing up in the small town of Medford, Oregon, I visibly stood out. I was different. With my dark olive skin and dark brown hair, I didn't look like anyone else. I fought for everything I got. But if I was passionate about something, nothing stood in my way. And even as a little girl, I dreamed of being a star. My parents always told me that I could do anything, and I believed them. My goal was to get out of Oregon and *be somebody*. For twenty years, I persevered, pushing through rejection and tough times. My faith never faltered.

Over the years, in my quest for the key to true happiness, I've read a library's worth of self-help books, starting with *The Power of Positive Thinking* and *The Road Less Traveled*. I have explored various spiritual practices. I saw a therapist for eleven years, long after the relationship had served its usefulness. Yet I never found the key.

I knew my problems were small compared to the problems of millions of others. But you can only walk in the shoes you're in, and these shoes weren't just hurting me; they were affecting my marriage and my family. How could I take care of them if I couldn't take care of myself? What kind of example was I setting for my daughters?

I had to admit to myself that the funk was largely all my own doing; that I was the problem. I've always been one who believes that if you can identify the problem, you can fix it. Or alternatively you can stick your head in the sand and vainly hope it will go away. Obviously, it wasn't going to go away on its own.

Finally, my "never quit" gene kicked in. I realized I had to fix myself first, and then I'd be able to tackle the rest of the dissatisfaction in my life. And where, you ask, did I start? By learning how to give a lap dance! Yes, a lap dancing class changed my life—it reconnected me to my sexuality and forced me to let go of my inhibitions. I got my mojo back and then some, and my husband got the old (along with the new and improved) Lisa back. Suddenly I was no longer self-conscious about my body. I picked up some new bedroom tricks, and dusted off some oldies but goodies (much, much more on this in the sex chapter). Needless to say, we were both pretty happy campers.

I discovered that I had the power to change anything in my life. Instead of sitting around feeling sorry for myself, and potentially losing my husband, I did something about it. This was the first step in renewing the life I wanted, one in which I looked and felt my best.

Also around that time, a lifetime of reading self-help books finally clicked. Reading *The Secret* was an important key. Even though I was familiar with many versions of its core philosophies, this time I was ready for the message and really embraced it. As the Buddhists say, "When the student is ready, the teacher will appear." I learned that all our thoughts are really just self-fulfilling prophecies. It didn't matter what I *did*, it was how I *felt* and *thought* about it. The negative self-talk and thoughts I had engaged in most of my life were what had been holding me back. Simplistic as this may sound, allowing myself to be open and consciously trying to stay positive all the time and be proactive worked for me big-time. I felt confident, in control, and lo and behold, *happy* for the first time in my life. Now I know this might sound too easy, but trust me, it's work and you have to be diligent.

I had experienced what I call a *Rinnavation*, a way to make a change and reboot my life by opening myself up to new possibilities, opportunities, and experiences. A Rinnavation is when you realize you want to change your life and you're committed to making it happen. It can start with a baby step, like taking a five-minute walk every day to kick-start an exercise routine, or a leap, like starting a business. Regardless of how you choose to embark on your own Rinnavation, the root cause is always the same—you acknowledge that something is a little (or a lot) off in your life, and you resolve to do something to start pulling yourself up out of the rut.

Rinnavation is, simply put, about looking your best, feeling your best, and doing your best, at every age and stage of life. We all have times in our lives when we feel just the opposite. You've packed on a few pounds, your social life is nonexistent, you hate your job, or something you can't even put your finger on is holding you back. I am a firm believer in action when this happens—whenever I have hit a roadblock in my life, doing something, anything, gets me on track to finding the solution. After all, you can't hit a moving target. And whether it is diet or exercise, starting a beauty routine, or changing your hairstyle, sometimes the *littlest* thing can make a huge difference. Even just by changing your thoughts, you can change your life. The key is, the change always starts with a positive outlook—sure, something isn't quite clicking, but you're going to start fixing it right now—and it often leads to much more than you originally set out to accomplish.

Getting my mojo back was just the beginning of a domino effect. I opened my first Belle Gray store in 2002 and then expanded to a second location in 2004. I was offered *Dancing with the Stars* in 2006. The following year, I starred in *Chicago* on Broadway. Who would have ever thought? I had never sung or danced professionally in my life! That same year, I was hired as the red-carpet commentator for the TV Guide Network. Since then I never look back. I look *forward* to every day because I have put my goals out there into the universe, and keep reaching for them. I'm always looking for the next Rinnavation.

I've never publicly discussed many of the personal details you'll read in the pages to follow. I'm sharing them with you now because the process of writing this book made me realize that all of these things—the good and the bad—are pieces of the puzzle, my puzzle, and I had to lay out all the pieces in order to see the bigger picture and what would work for me. Don't worry—I won't be getting all New Age on you. Positive thinking alone can't make you lose weight and get fit, nor will it give you a great haircut or fabulous style. These are the other pieces of the puzzle, but everything's connected. To look great you have to feel great, and vice versa. I've spent decades experimenting with every beauty, diet, exercise, and fashion regimen there is. What I've learned could fill a library (and what I've spent experimenting could sustain an entire bank). Since you probably barely have time to read this book, I have distilled just the best stuff, enough to get you on track for your own Rinnavation.

You may be seeking to revamp your appearance through diet, exercise, or a new beauty routine. I've been there. It is part of my job to look good at all times whether I like it or not, and this is especially true when I am in front of the camera. But I don't wake up every morning looking red-carpet ready. Far from it! Sometimes my face looks like a pizza because I have so many zits, I feel bloated, or my skin looks less than sun-kissed. Through the years, I've perfected the secrets to looking my best in the least amount of time—I've had to in order to survive in this business! I've culled information from the top hair stylists, makeup artists, exercise gurus, doctors, and fashion stylists, and I'm ready to pass it along. I've been so lucky to work with amazing people, but the truth is that anyone can do these, without a team of experts, and with minimal cost and time.

You might be trying to refocus your life on something you love. I know what that's like, too. Over the years, through will and necessity, I've learned to make my personal passions the driving forces of my life: fashion, fitness, marriage, sex, motherhood, dancing, and spirituality. Realizing these passions in the first place is what keeps me focused and motivated. Fortunately, I have been able to channel these passions, both personally and professionally, into things that are real and lasting, and very satisfying. For example, I took my passion for clothes and my addiction to shopping and opened my boutique line, Belle Gray, with my husband, Harry (who built the stores with his bare hands, I might add!).

I know firsthand that women have just too few hours in the day and that in the hectic whirlwind of our lives, looking fabulous is usually way down on the list of priorities. Who *ever* has enough time to accomplish everything they set out to do in a day? Getting the kids fed and to school on time is where the energy and precious minutes tend to go. But then, suddenly, something comes along that forces you to make the time to focus on yourself. Whether it's your high school reunion, your wedding (or someone else's), or fitting into those skinny jeans for the weekend, you need to look your best—fast.

Believe it or not, it is possible to make a real transformation in as little as a week. Many of my tricks are *trompe l'oeil*—little things that trick the eye into making you look thinner, fitter, more glowing. I will guide you step by step, from day one to day seven. I have tried hundreds of these strategies over the years and have learned which ones work, which ones don't work, and most importantly, which ones work quickly. I have included only the ones I know are the best—the most effective and the fastest.

Whenever I meet someone new, they unfailingly ask me one of three questions (sometimes all three!). In no particular order, they are: Who cuts your hair? How do you keep your body looking like that? How do you balance it all? Answering these questions was the original impetus for writing this book. Now, I am no expert, but I wanted to share my secrets for looking great, feeling great, and doing great. But a funny thing happened along the way. As I started writing the book, I began flashing back on my life and experiences, and I started seeing patterns in my life that I had never noticed before. I could track my evolution through the decades, through the exercise, fashion, and relationships I was involved in at the time. A lot of it wasn't pretty, but at the end of the day,

I was proud of how far I'd come, and grateful for both my triumphs and my failures. It all made me who I am today, and I don't regret any of it. I can honestly say that I'm enjoying the best time of my life—professionally, personally, physically, sexually, and emotionally. Hey, it only took four decades! But it's never too late to start working toward *your* best life.

I'll give you tips to help you transform yourself so you can look and feel great, sometimes in a very short amount of time; but this is more than just a quick fix, a "how to get into your skinny jeans by Friday" kind of book. Yes, that's part of it, but there is a far bigger message. I often joke that I am on a mission—to help women get out of their comfort zones, to take a risk, to experience their own "Dancing with the Stars moment." I see women who are overweight, or out of shape, who seem to have given up. A lot of this stems from the fact that we women don't take time for ourselves. We are constantly only doing for others at our jobs and at home. We don't feel entitled to do things just for ourselves. Often that leads us into a big rut. I firmly believe that anyone can change their lives for the better, and it needn't be something major. Remember, we are multitaskers extraordinaire. We can do anything. And even the smallest change can take you in the right direction toward your own Rinnavation. You just have to make up your mind to make it happen. Whether it's taking a walk around the block, spicing up your sex life, or having a spa day with your girlfriends, it's about doing something just for you. You might feel a little guilty at first, but you will find that these little changes will benefit everyone around you. You can't make others feel good if you don't feel good about yourself. I really believe it is that basic.

It's all about doing what you need to do to be your best self. We have to be realistic and work with what we have. Let's face it, none of us will ever have Pamela Anderson's body or Angelina Jolie's face. But if you really work with what you have, you'll be amazed at how you look and feel, and how others respond to you.

The tips and routines in this book are easy to do, because if it's too hard you won't do it. And I will save you from many mistakes by sharing some of my blunders. You can cherry-pick the things that appeal to you and leave the rest. If you hate exercise, start with a few diet and beauty tips. One baby step at a time. If it feels good, take another step. If it doesn't, take a step back, and try something else—a different hairstyle or a new outfit. Have fun with it—what's the worst that can happen?

As you begin your transformation, try not to overthink it. It's easy to come up with all the reasons not to do something—no time, no money, no willpower—but it's just as easy to get up and do it. What are you waiting for?

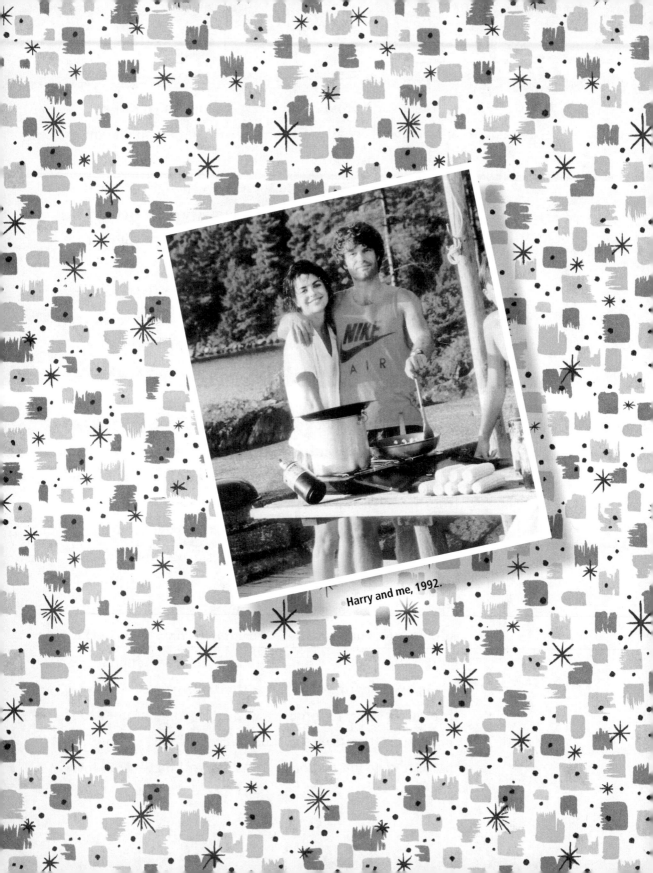

Harry and me, 1992.

CHAPTER ONE

HEALTH INSIDE OUT

I've never been a dieter. Because I exercise regularly, and eat small portions of healthy foods throughout the day, I never have a lot of extra pounds to lose. But when I was pregnant with my first daughter, Delilah, I packed on thirty-two pounds, and after I gave birth, they weren't coming off as fast as I would have liked. All the rage then was the Atkins diet, and it sounded easy enough: eat huge portions of meat and other proteins. I threw myself into the diet, like I do everything else, gorging on pork rinds, forty-ounce steaks, and heavy cream.

Not only did I not lose one single pound, but I also developed a wicked case of constipation. I didn't poop for two weeks! I felt like a big, greasy, smelly tub of lard. Totally gross! Add to that the always attractive state of ketosis, during which, I found out later, your body is burning fat and emitting acetone gases. A nutritionist told me she could always tell when someone was on the Atkins diet because of the smell—your breath and body smell like rotting flesh. Attractive! To make matters worse, Harry went on the diet, and he dropped pounds instantly.

It took me months to get my body back to normal, functionwise, and that was the last diet for me. Extremes in anything never work for me, so I have to go about losing weight sensibly. Though it took four months to lose the baby weight, it was worth it, and within a year I had my body back in the shape it had been before my pregnancy (I believe it takes a full year to really get your body back after the baby).

Like death and taxes, diets are an unpleasant fact of life. Every season it seems there is some new fad diet or twist on an old one—low-carb, low-fat, low-calorie, you name it. In general, I am not a big believer in diets, because in the long run they just don't work. Then, when you fall off, which you eventually do, you gain back the weight you lost and sometimes more. I am, however, a fan of short-term "mini-diets" because there is a light at the end of the tunnel.

As a rule, I am a pretty healthy eater. Basically, if I know it's not good for me, I try to stay away from it. That means all processed white foods (bad carbs), such as white sugar, white rice, and white flour. I also try to avoid fried foods. Instead of counting calories, I stick to foods I know have nutritional value—vegetables, fruits, and lean proteins. I find it easier if I have a set list of foods that I can eat every day. Not only do I not have to think about it (that time factor again), but I don't have to count calories or points, measure, or brush up on my math to come up with the right combination of fats, protein, and carbs.

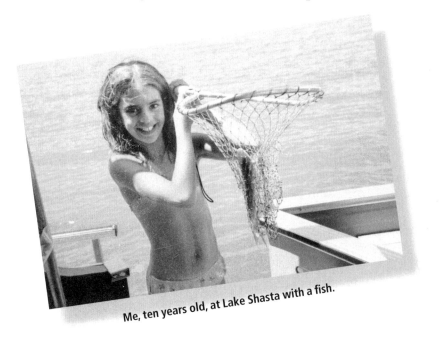

Me, ten years old, at Lake Shasta with a fish.

A few diet plans work really well for me. One, which I found in a book called *The Blood Type Diet*, recommends choosing foods by your blood type. I am a Type O, and according to *The Blood Type Diet*, if I eat a lot of red meat, protein, and fewer carbs, the weight just drops off. This eating plan is not as extreme as Atkins, and though it works for me, everyone's body (and blood type) is different. I have a friend who swears by the *BBDO* diet—no bread, booze, desserts, and off comes the weight. I don't think anyone can eat pasta or drink alcohol every day and lose weight. Not going to happen. Alcohol is wasted calories; it bloats you and makes you fat, period. I love a good glass of wine but, if I'm really trying to slim down, I limit myself to one glass a week. I also believe in having one day a week where I let myself have whatever I want, so I don't feel deprived. Then the next day I get back on track.

When I was pregnant with both my daughters, I had Zone meals delivered to me, not because I wanted to lose weight but because I wanted to eat a healthy and balanced diet. This way I didn't have to think about it (or God forbid, cook). In my twenties, I discovered the Fit for Life diet plan, and I've followed the principles of food combining ever since. The basic principle is you don't mix carbohydrates and proteins in the same meal. I have fruit in the morning, protein and vegetables for lunch, and carbs and veggies for dinner. My diet is a healthy smorgasbord!

Another key component of my diet is eating small portions throughout the day. I've always watched my mom and she has never dieted in her life. And she's always weighed between 110 and 113 pounds—she never fluctuates beyond that range (good genes, lucky for me!). She eats small portions of healthy foods, enjoys desserts, and never binges. (It's hard to believe, I know, but it's true.) I firmly believe that one of the reasons Americans are overweight is because of the huge portions we are served. It's like a Thanksgiving feast every night. When you eat a huge meal, your stomach stretches. When you begin to eat smaller portions, your stomach starts to shrink, so you don't need to eat as much to feel full. I call it the natural "gastric bypass" diet. If I order food out, I eat half of the portion, wrap the other half, and take it with me for later. Since it takes about twenty minutes for your brain to tell your stomach you're full, I try to eat slowly, and find that these small meals, consumed at a slow pace, satisfy me so that I don't have cravings. I guarantee that if you try eating small portions and eating more slowly for three weeks, you will lose weight. Each portion should be about two to three ounces, the size of the palm of your hand. It works because it's easy—no counting calories, and you eat what you and your body want.

Throughout the day, I will have little snacks. My favorites are a handful of almonds, a stick of string cheese, an apple with a tablespoon of peanut butter, a piece of cheddar cheese, or a scoop of Nutella and a scoop of peanut butter.

By the Clock

It's important to eat every three hours or so, as your blood sugar starts to drop. Eating often throughout the day also speeds up your metabolism and keeps you from gorging (or being a hungry, raging bitch!). *When you eat is as important as what you eat.* Eating six small meals rather than three big meals helps you lose weight fast, because you stay full and don't have the blood sugar crashes that cause cravings and overeating, so you are less likely to binge. As many of us have discovered the hard way, starving yourself not only makes you grumpy and tired, but actually prevents you from losing weight! Not eating, or skipping a meal, actually slows metabolism. Your body goes into "starvation mode" and begins to conserve and store the calories and fat you've consumed, instead of burning them. So keep that furnace stoked and burning all day long.

I don't believe you have to eat a hugely varied diet if you don't want to. I eat the same things over and over. Again, keep it simple. Eat what you like; just eat it in small portions and try to make your choices as healthy as possible. I also eat only if I'm hungry; so much of when we eat is tied to our emotions, and I avoid those traps by keeping busy. I'll go for a walk, or do something around the house, if I feel compelled to needlessly snack. Get busy—you will forget you are hungry.

Food and How You Look

Who doesn't want clear, radiant skin? Fewer wrinkles? Fewer pimples? Unfortunately, you can't stop the aging process (yet), but there are many things you can do to make it look like you have. Working with my doctor, who specializes in alternative medicine, I have developed a regimen of vitamin supplements combined with diet and exercise that truly turn back the clock. They give you energy, improve your memory (perfect for that high school reunion!), reduce water bloat, curb cravings, build lean muscle, make your skin glow and hair shine, and regulate hormones.

The human body is an amazing machine, but like the finest Maserati, it performs optimally only when it has the right fuel. Nature (another amazing "machine") has provided this fuel in a bunch of super or power foods, what I call my Fab Foods. They really should be called the perfect foods because they are loaded with fiber, vitamins, minerals, and protein, and have fat-burning, metabolism-boosting properties and hardly any calories and fat; plus they taste really good! Not only are they filling, but they sneakily speed up your metabolism, flush out toxins and excess fluids, tone your skin, and make your hair and skin glow!

It is as simple as eating a short list of certain foods every day. My rule of thumb is, the more colorful they are, the better they are for you. The best part is that most of them require no cooking! Since (true confession time) I'm not much of a cook, I find these foods especially brilliant because they require very little preparation time and no complicated recipes. Lose weight *and* save time—you gotta love it!

When it comes to diet and nutrition, a lot of what actually works is good old common sense and what we've been told all along—eat more fruits and vegetables; stay away from processed foods and starchy, "bad" carbs; eat smaller meals throughout the day. My diet philosophy is all of the above, plus, *it must be easy, time-efficient, and great-tasting.* The plans I've developed satisfy all of these criteria. It works for me, and I think it can work for you if you give it a chance. After all, what do you have to lose, besides weight, fatigue, dull skin and hair, wrinkles, and other battle scars of aging?

If you eat these foods every day for a week, you can achieve amazing results without breaking a sweat. (We'll get to that part in the exercise chapter.) And who knows, since this isn't really a "diet," you might just find yourself sticking with it, or at the very least picking up a few lifelong habits. And if you fall off the wagon and eat junk foods with the kids, don't beat yourself up. Just start again the next day. I do it all the time! I mean, life without pizza and ice cream is just plain dull!

FAB FOODS

These are my must-have foods. I eat as many of them as I can every day. It helps that I love them, so it's a treat, not a chore.

Berries: raspberries, blueberries, cranberries, blackberries, anything with the word "berry" at the end of it. They have tons of vitamins C and E, fiber, and antioxidants. The fiber fills you up, curbs cravings, and helps eliminate toxins and fluids. The antioxidants give you glowing skin, shiny hair, and strong nails. They also improve memory and brain function (good for remembering names at that special event!).

Yogurt: it's full of calcium (400 mg. per cup), which has been proven to help burn fat and promote weight loss, plus protein (8 grams per cup), which helps your body build muscle. One cup has as much potassium as a banana. Potassium flushes out sodium, ridding you of fluids and bloat. It also contains lecithin, which helps digestion. Yogurt also contains probiotics that strengthen the immune system, and friendly bacteria, which break down toxins and help your body absorb more vitamins, minerals, and proteins. Make sure you read the labels carefully and choose only those that have live and active cultures, and no added sugar or high-fructose corn syrup.

Oats and whole grains: oatmeal, barley, oat bran, brown rice, rye, and quinoa are a perfect combo of fiber, protein, and complex carbs. They are also rich in magnesium and potassium. Fiber curbs cravings and speeds metabolism, so having a bowl of oatmeal for breakfast will keep you full throughout the morning. Sprinkle on some cinnamon, which will keep you from reaching for a sugary, mid-morning snack.

Spinach: it is full of B_6 vitamins, fiber, protein (who knew?), calcium, lecithin, vitamins A, C, K, iron, and coenzyme COQ. It also has magnesium, which helps your body absorb vitamin D, and prevents fatigue and depression. The majority of women have seriously low levels of vitamin D, which can mean serious trouble for your bones. I suffer from low bone density so I am very vigilant about getting enough vitamin D and calcium. Spinach has a high water content, which is great for flushing out toxins and excess fluids. Chlorophyll speeds slimming by helping heal and detox the liver so it can break down and flush out toxins. Goodbye, bloat!

Legumes/beans: chickpeas, kidney, pinto, red, and black beans have huge amounts of protein and fiber. Beans block the enzyme that turns carbs to sugar, preventing blood sugar levels from spiking, which leads to fat storage. The protein strengthens collagen and elastin, the tissue that keeps your skin looking firm and healthy. I eat just 3 cups a week (canned are fine) to get all these amazing benefits.

Eggs: they have zinc, protein, amino acids, B vitamins, which build white blood cells, and antibodies to fight off illness. Just two eggs eliminate fat-soluble toxins. Don't ignore the yolk—it has all the nutrients—lutein, choline, vitamins A, D, E, and B_6. Try to buy the ones that come from pastured hens, or are enriched to provide double or triple amounts of omega 3 fatty acids, vitamin E, and vitamin A.

Asparagus: it's got amazing diuretic properties. Try to eat eight spears a day with 64 ounces of water for one week to flush out toxins and excess fluids, and to reduce bloat.

Broccoli: it's easy to find and inexpensive, and is chock-full of vitamins A and C, calcium, potassium, folic acid, and fiber.

Nuts and seeds: These are true superfoods, and there are so many varieties to choose from: almonds, pecans, pistachios, walnuts, sunflower seeds, flaxseeds, peanuts, and peanut butter. They contain omega 3 fatty acids, magnesium, potassium, vitamins B_6 and E, and soluble fiber. Fiber helps stabilize blood sugar and prevents insulin surges and weight gain. I always carry nuts with me and eat them every day.

Healthy oils: olive, canola, and flaxseed. These contain good fats and are a great source of vitamin E, and are better for you than vegetable oils, which are more difficult to digest and can lead to inflammation.

Chocolate: when I'm feeling hormonal, I crave sweets, especially chocolate. It turns out that chocolate not only satisfies my sweet tooth but also produces "feel good" endorphins in the brain. Try to choose brands that have a 70 percent or greater cocoa content, as these have less sugar and more of the beneficial ingredients.

Other foods I eat all the time—especially when I need a quick snack—include bananas, popcorn, and apples with peanut butter.

DYNAMITE DRINKS

Water: the perfect beverage. Drink a minimum of eight glasses of water a day. The benefits are proven: drinking water increases metabolism, reduces hunger, burns fat, and flushes toxins from your body.

You should always drink a glass of water as soon as you wake up. It jump-starts your metabolism and begins flushing toxins. Room-temperature water is best—add a little lemon or cranberry or pomegranate juice to liven it up. Lemon juice reduces bloat and helps detox, cranberry juice flushes toxins, and pomegranate is full of antioxidants and energizers. I continue to drink water throughout the day, with or without the added lemon, cranberry, or pomegranate juice.

The Waker-Upper

I find that the best waker-upper is water with lemon zest and lemon juice. Lemon zest improves liver detox and speeds fat metabolism, and this beverage is really refreshing. Combine the juice of half a lemon with 1 teaspoon of freshly grated zest and add to 12 ounces of room temperature water.

Green tea: I love green tea! It boosts metabolism to burn calories and has tons of antioxidants. I drink iced green tea with stevia throughout the day. Yerba maté tea is great, too. I start my day with a cup or two, sweetened with stevia, every morning. Other super teas include dandelion root and milk thistle teas, which detox and flush the liver.

Smoothies: here are a few of my favorites: Blend 1 cup frozen blueberries, $\frac{1}{2}$ cup pomegranate juice, 2 cups apple juice, 6 oz. soft tofu, and $\frac{1}{2}$ frozen banana. Delicious. Also tasty: Combine 1 cup frozen berries, 1 banana, 1 cup non-fat, no-sugar yogurt, $\frac{1}{2}$ cup orange juice, and low-fat milk or soy milk. Blend until creamy. And, last but not least, a truly decadent one: Combine half of a banana, a cup of chocolate Silk soy milk, 4 ice cubes, and 1 tablespoon of peanut butter. Blend together and swoon.

Liver Detox

Learning about the importance of the liver was life-changing for me. The liver is the engine that keeps the body running on max by controlling detoxification, energy, and weight, and is responsible for processing alcohol, sugar, and fat. An overstressed liver can't burn fat and convert food into energy efficiently. Cleansing the liver of toxins revs metabolism by 23 percent, allowing the liver to eliminate toxins, fluids, and fats. Your liver affects every aspect of your appearance—your hair, nails, skin, weight, *everything*.

I knew the liver was important for overall health and well-being, but it wasn't until I did a three-day spa detox that I became a disciple of the liver detox program. Last summer, after a grueling schedule shooting my fourth cardio ballroom

DVD in three day's time (among many other things), I was drained, physically and emotionally, and I needed to detox and decompress, so my friend Jana and I booked a weekend spa retreat in Palm Springs. For three days, we consumed fourteen different juices a day, accompanied by yoga, massage, meditation, and colonics. While some people love the results but hate the process (the colonics) of these types of retreats, I loved everything about it. I lost three pounds in three days. I had two colonics and two fabulous massages and a lemon salt body scrub, and it made me feel like a new woman. For me, it's a great way to drop weight quickly and to recharge and rejuvenate. I absolutely adored it!

The liquid diet at the spa consisted of a range of drinks with spirulina, wheatgrass, barley, acidophilus, freshly squeezed vegetable juice, lemon water, enzymes, liver and kidney-purifying teas, and blood-purifying tea. They were amazing. While you might not be able to get to a top-notch spa anytime soon, here are some cleansing drinks you can make at home:

Cleansing lemonade: combine 2 tablespoons of freshly squeezed lemon or lime juice, 1 tablespoon of pure maple syrup, a dash of cayenne pepper, and 8 ounces of water. Drink before breakfast and lunch. This is an amazing anti-inflammatory that reduces bloating and puffiness.

Super energy drink: combine 1 cup soy milk, a banana, 2 to

3 teaspoons of spirulina, 1 cup of berries, half a cup of yogurt, and a cup of pomegranate juice. Blend, drink, and feel instantly energized.

Vegetable or chicken broth: drink a cup of this before meals to curb your appetite and add to your water intake.

Liquid salad: no time to eat, never mind cook? Drink an 8-ounce glass of vegetable juice mixed with 2 tablespoons of green superfood powder sold in health food stores. The powder contains chlorophyll, which neutralizes toxins, flushes out excess water, and speeds fat metabolism.

I also love the Miracle Juice Detox that Anna Louise Gittelman includes in *The Fat Flush Plan.*

PREPARED DRINKS AND MIXES

Satiatrim: this blend of safflower oil, sunflower oil, soy protein, and calcium triggers a protein that makes you feel full for up to four hours.

Borba skin balance water: this fortified water contains a bio-vitamin complex with a scientifically designed blend of nutrients. High in antioxidant vitamins C and E, with four essential B vitamins, this wonder drink is aspartame-free, sodium-free, and has zero calories and zero grams of carbohydrates. The Pomegranate, Açai Berry, Lychee Fruit, and Guanábana Fruit flavors are surprisingly tasty.

FOOD SUPPLEMENTS

You can fulfill most of your daily vitamin and mineral requirements by simply eating the foods I've listed in this chapter, but there are some supplements that do aid in burning fat, speeding up metabolism, and detoxing. Bear in mind that these supplements can have side effects, so you should consult your doctor or health practitioner before using these or any other supplements. (Remember, I'm no expert. These are just some things that I've found useful.)

Kyo-Green powder: this is one of my favorite supplements. It's a blend of barley and wheat grasses, chlorella, brown rice, and kelp. You mix it with juice, and it gives you all your vitamins and minerals and tons of energy. You can buy the powder at any health or whole food store.

SoCal Cleanse: this is a supplement that combines natural detoxifying compounds like milk thistle with metabolism-boosting ingredients such as green tea capsules. Some celebrities have reported losing twenty pounds in a month by using it.

Spirulina, or blue green algae, is something else I recommend. Spirulina consists of plant proteins that contain chlorophyll, beta-carotene, protein, antioxidants,

B-complex vitamins, and all the essential fatty acids. It comes in many forms—capsules, powder, or liquid.

Chromium; vitamin D: (particularly vitamin D_3, which is absorbed three to five times more effectively than other D vitamins); **magnesium** (which helps activate the vitamin D); and **calcium** daily are also highly recommended. These all help speed up metabolism and keep your body revved.

Miracle Reds Powder: this has a great fruity taste and contains omega 3 fatty acids to burn fat. A blend of nutrient-rich, anti-aging anti-oxidants, polyphenols, and heart-friendly plant sterols, the powder contains an abundant source of hand-selected anti-oxidants that support cell activity and fight free radicals.

Another of my personal favorites are the vitamin gummy bears from Borba, called **Gummy Bear Boosters,** which taste like candy but contain a laundry list of vitamins, minerals, and other nutrients, and are great for your skin.

SUPER HERBS AND SPICES

Consider adding these to your foods. They have no calories, boost flavor, and help speed weight loss.

Cayenne pepper: this speeds up fat-burning and adds zest to food, and it helps you detox by clearing out mucus and other excess fluids. It can also be used as a pain reliever and decongestant.

Red pepper: it contains vitamin A, supplies energy, boosts immunity, and relieves pain.

Cinnamon: it's an anti-inflammatory and contains calcium, magnesium, and fiber. It helps reduce cravings by stabilizing blood sugar. Apple-cinnamon tea is especially yummy.

Oregano: it has fiber, and vitamins A, C, and K.

Basil: it has vitamin K and flavonoids. It protects cells, functions as an anti-inflammatory, and is an immunity booster.

Mint: this contains vitamins A and C, as well as fiber and iron. It's a great flavor booster, muscle relaxant, allergy-easer, and stomach-soother.

THE BIG NO-NO'S

Avoid these foods like the plague:

- Anything that contains a lot of sodium
- Soda—even diet soda bloats you
- Processed foods
- Bad carbs—white flour, white pasta, white rice, sugar
- Artificial sweeteners

MY DOWNFALLS

I have a wicked sweet tooth, especially when I'm feeling hormonal, so these are the foods I try to avoid during these times: Nestle Tollhouse Cookie Dough, cookies, cake, blueberry pie that Harry makes. I also have a soft spot for nachos (who doesn't?), and red velvet cupcakes. Figure out your no-no's and save them for a special occasion!

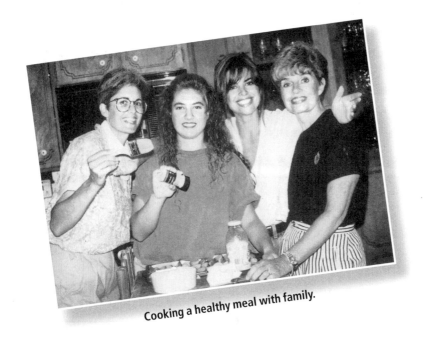

Cooking a healthy meal with family.

How to Eat Healthy as a Family

Maintaining a healthy diet with two young kids and a husband who doesn't really have to worry about watching what he eats is hard, but you can do it. It just takes pre-planning a lot of the time. Often, when I'm being a stickler about my diet, I'll prepare my own food for dinner, the girls will eat Sloppy Joes, and Harry will have a steak and a salad. Hey, just because your husband and kids want one thing for dinner doesn't mean you have to eat it! Steam some veggies or have a salad with a grilled piece of chicken or other fun add-ins, like blueberries and nuts—you're cooking anyway, so what's one more dish? As I mentioned earlier, of course you're going to fall off the wagon and eat junk food with the kids every so often, but maintaining your own program as often as possible is important. And of course eating healthy meals together as a family is so important; but let's face it, there are a lot of Sloppy Joe nights when you're a busy mom.

My "Fit into Your Favorite Jeans by Friday" Plan

When I am trying to lose weight and detox fast, or just want to kick-start my metabolism and boost my energy level, I do one to three days of the cleansing drinks, along with smoothies and juices; and then, over the next week, I add in small, healthy, slimming mini-meals every three hours. It releases toxins and cleans me out, and I get immediate results and feel great!

I'll supplement this plan with Nikki Haskell's Star-Caps; they speed up your metabolism and work like a charm before a big event. I also eat Goji berries for energy and drink lots of yerba maté tea and green tea. Another great pick-me-up is Emergen-C Super Energy Booster packets. I also love Gaia herbs, especially their Diet Slim and Sound Sleep liquid capsules.

Here is a sample of my seven-day fast-and-detox meal plan that'll have you fitting into your favorite jeans by Friday. You will see that it is not rigid or full of rules or combinations. In fact, I encourage you to make up your own recipes and combinations. You really can't go wrong if you stick to these foods and drinks, and remember: You gotta "eat clean" in order to have a rockin' body—that means no processed foods!

Day 1: I drink Miracle Juice or special lemonade as instructed on page 27.

Days 2 and 3: I supplement the detox drinks with smoothies and light meals that include the Fab Foods above.

Seven-Day Detox Meal Plan

BREAKFAST

Rule of Thumb: breakfast should be your biggest good-carb meal. I choose oatmeal, whole-grain or all-natural fiber cereals.

Water: start with an 8-oz. glass of water with lemon, the warmer the better. I also drink what I call my "happy tea" every day—green tea or yerba maté tea, sweetened with stevia, a natural sweetener (I don't use any artificial sweeteners).

1 cup oatmeal made with water or low-fat milk: (I use soy or almond milk because I'm allergic to cow's milk.) Top with berries, flaxseed, and cinnamon. You can sweeten it with stevia if you like.

Yogurt with berries and cinnamon: I get all the health benefits of yogurt and berries, plus the craving-reducing effects of the cinnamon. I mix 1 cup yogurt (sugar-free) with any or all of the toppings from the fab foods list—berries, flaxseeds, nuts, no-sugar-added muesli, cinnamon, dark or semi-sweet chocolate chips.

Drink water, water, and more water.

MID-MORNING SNACK

Pick one and enjoy it!

A protein or power bar: I always carry these in my bag for between-meal snacks.

A handful of almonds: (about 10–15), washed down with 8 ounces of any of the cleansing beverages. (I also carry these with me at all times.)

A sliced apple: dipped in peanut butter.

Green tea: one cup (hot or iced) with stevia.

LUNCH

Rule of Thumb: Lunch should center on lean proteins and vitamin-and-mineral–packed vegetables. During the Detox Meal diet, though, I stick with beans. There is an endless variety of things you can do with beans. They should be the cornerstone of your lunch every day for the first week because the fiber will make you feel full, and the nutrients will rev up your metabolism so you keep burning fat throughout the day.

Three-bean chili is one of my lunch favorites. To make it, I sauté onions and peppers in olive oil, then add fresh or canned tomatoes and continue to sauté until the tomatoes are cooked through. Then I add in rinsed canned beans and pepper (white, black, or cayenne) to taste and cook on medium low heat until the beans are cooked through and the flavors have melded, about thirty minutes. Serve the chili in a bowl and top it with a dollop of plain reduced-fat or fat-free yogurt.

Other combos I like are:

1 cup canned black beans: drained and heated. Add plain yogurt on top, and avocado on the side.

1 can of white kidney (cannellini) beans: drained. Mix with chopped tomato and onion to taste. No cooking required!

1 pound green beans: washed and snapped. Place in a microwave-safe container, cover with plastic wrap, and heat for five minutes or until tender. Toss with 2 teaspoons olive oil and ½ teaspoon of garlic salt.

I always serve the beans with a side dish of brown rice, avocado, broccoli, or asparagus drizzled with lemon juice. And you should experiment with spices and herbs, like parsley, oregano, cinnamon, basil, rosemary. They add flavor and have fat-burning and detoxing properties.

If I'm on the go and can't prepare one of the dishes above, I often will stop at a local deli and order a salad. One of my favorites is spinach leaves, grilled onion, and chicken breast. It's healthy, and it hits the spot. Or I get an egg-white omelet with fat-free sour cream, Swiss cheese, and sliced avocado.

MID-AFTERNOON SNACK

Just like your morning snack, pick one and enjoy your energy boost!

Do It Yourself Trail Mix: mix together your favorite nuts (peanuts, soybeans, almonds, sunflower seeds) with dried fruits and a handful of dark or semi-sweet chocolate chips. Carry this with you and eat a handful when you feel hungry or sluggish. The fiber stabilizes your blood sugar and curbs carvings, and the nutrients give you energy.

Delicious Dip: combine avocados, tomatoes, lime or lemon juice, and yogurt. Mix to desired consistency and eat with veggies or whole grain crackers.

Hummus or salsa: store brands are fine if they are all-natural and have no sugar added. Both have little or no fat, and few calories. Pair them with veggies— carrots, celery, broccoli, or whole grain crackers or chips (no more than five or six), and you have a great appetizer or snack.

A cleansing drink: an 8-ounce glass.

Fiber charge: combine a tablespoon of Benefiber, or other fiber powder with a packet of Emergen-C and 8 ounces of water. This will give you an energy boost, curb cravings, and jump-start your digestion.

Green or oolong tea: one cup, hot or iced.

DINNER

Rule of Thumb: Dinner should be your lightest meal of the day. I choose fat-burning, metabolism-boosting foods that will keep my body churning straight through until morning. The perfect dinner is a light, low-sodium, broth-based soup and small leafy green salad. It will leave you feeling light and clean. And substituting an omelette packed with veggies for soup is a light and healthy choice as well.

Before dinner, I'll have a cleansing drink or some broth (vegetable or chicken). This takes the edge off my hunger before I sit down at the table. With dinner, I'll drink 8 ounces of water with a splash of cranberry or lemon juice.

Salad can be served as a side dish with soup or as the main course. I use uncooked, organic spinach leaves, and drizzle on 1 tablespoon red wine vinegar and 1 teaspoon olive oil. Or I make a raspberry dressing by blending $\frac{1}{2}$ cup raspberries, 3 tablespoons lemon juice, 1 tablespoon honey, and $\frac{1}{3}$ cup olive oil. Then I toss on some sunflower seeds, chickpeas, pistachios, whatever tickles my fancy. If it is my main course, I add other ingredients, like hard-boiled eggs, tomatoes, avocado, asparagus, broccoli, or carrots.

Sometimes I'll treat myself to a steak salad as a dinner entrée. I'll buy everything prepared—steak, brussels sprouts, grated parmesan cheese—from a healthy natural foods market like Trader Joe's, Whole Foods, or Erewhon; then at home I'll cut up the steak and mix it with lettuce, the cheese, brussels sprouts, and a light dressing of balsamic vinegar and olive oil. Here are a couple of my other main course favorites:

Dynamic dinner omelet: 2 egg whites, tomatoes, parmesan cheese, chives, herbs such as oregano, basil, or parsley, and any of the following Fab Foods: asparagus, mushrooms, spinach, peppers, onions.

Easy chicken soup: (even I can manage this):

2 cans chicken broth (low sodium). You can substitute vegetable broth if you don't eat meat.

1 large can whole or chopped tomatoes

1 can no-sugar-added beans—name your flavor: pinto, cannellini, green, kidney, soy, or butter beans or lentils.

4 carrots, chopped

½ stalk chopped celery with leaves

½ teaspoon black pepper

⅛ teaspoon white pepper (or cayenne pepper for a flavor boost and to rev metabolism)

1 large onion, quartered

¼ teaspoon basil

Combine all ingredients in a large soup pan and cook on medium heat. Bring to a boil, and then reduce heat to medium low. Cover and cook for thirty minutes.

Optional: add chunks of cooked chicken for flavor.

EVENING SNACK

You guessed it: select one and savor it!

1 cup non-caffeinated tea such as dandelion root or milk thistle (which cleanses the liver) will usually satisfy me. If you desire (though you probably won't because you will feel so sated from dinner), have a snack (but never after 8 P.M.!) of:

½ cup of berries or an ounce of dark chocolate or a handful of nuts

Sugar-free Popsicles or Dreyer's Frozen Fruit Bars are also two of my favorite no-guilt pleasures.

I also like sugar-free Jell-O cups (topped with Cool Whip if I need a little something more). Each cup is just ten calories, and satisfies my need for something sweet. I'll make it myself too—my mom used to make us Jell-O salad every night using a different flavor and mixing in fresh fruit, and now I make Jell-O with my daughters. It's easy for them to do and really fun, not to mention great for when I'm trying to stay in red-carpet shape. (I enjoy it so much, I even did a commercial for Jell-O years ago!)

AND FINALLY . . .

Before bed, drink eight ounces of lemon water. Then give yourself a pat on the back. Not only have you fulfilled (exceeded, actually) your daily requirement of water, you have also fueled your body so that it is now on autopilot, fully functioning like a fine machine. Sleep soundly while your body is busy burning fat and calories, building muscle, and cleansing your liver.

Copy the list of Fab Foods and the list of Dynamite Drinks, and carry them around with you. I find it easiest to buy everything on the list in one fell swoop; then you always have them on hand. You can't eat and drink them if you don't have them in your kitchen. Create a game where you see how many of these foods you can eat a day. And, of course, enjoy!

Super-Quick Fix—Look Great in Three Days.

As I mentioned, when I need to drop a few pounds quickly, or fit into a gown for a special event, I do a fasting detox for one to three days, during which I drink the teas, juices, and smoothies I've outlined. I'll also eat pureed vegetable soups, but no solids—if I'm really serious I do only liquids for three days. But even just *one* day can clean out the toxins and get your skin glowing. (Remember, you should consult with your physician before implementing any new diet or exercise program, including a detox.) Detoxification gets rid of water bloat, puffiness, and toxins, and refreshes and revives your skin, hair, and body. I cut out *all* white food, processed food, sugar, alcohol, and salt three weeks before an event. I know a liquid diet isn't for everybody, but I am telling you what works for me, and if you try my super-quick fix—or even a variation of it—and it works, then I know your body will look amazing in your dress.

That, in a nutshell, is my diet plan. In the next chapter, I will show you how to combine quick, easy exercises to speed up your metabolism and boost your self-esteem even more. Get those skinny jeans ready!

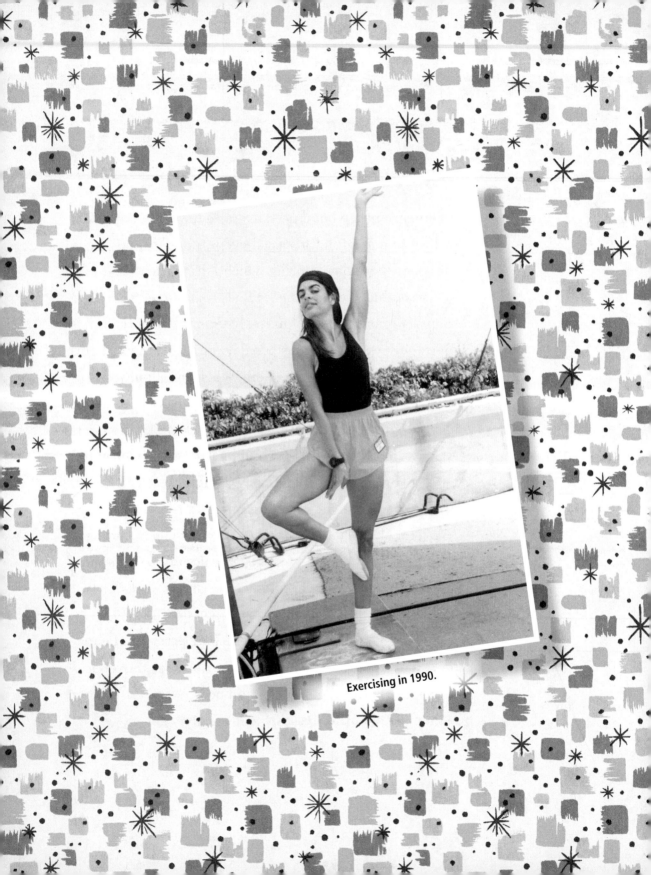

Exercising in 1990.

CHAPTER TWO

MOVE WHAT
YOU'VE GOT

If we just danced every day, we'd all be happy.

—RITA WILSON

A few years back, I was approached to appear on the first season of a new show called *Dancing with the Stars*. I had never sung or danced professionally in my life, but I had always been an exercise fanatic and was in pretty good shape. I love to dance at weddings and other celebrations, and I thought what a great crash course on really learning how to dance participating in the show would be. There was also the terrifying prospect of dancing (and possibly making a fool of myself) in front of twenty million people, but despite that, my gut said "go for it." My agents, however, were dead-set against it. They were afraid the show would tank, and it would somehow hurt my career. So reluctantly, I turned it down.

When *Dancing with the Stars* became a monster hit in its first season, I wanted to kick myself for turning it down, and not trusting my instincts. A few months after the show's debut, I was at my 8:15 A.M. Saturday spinning class, when out of the corner of my eye I saw Andrea Wong, the head of alternative programming at ABC. She was the executive who had brought *DWTS* to the United States from England. She took a huge risk in convincing the ABC executives to do this show, and, in doing so, gave the network a huge boost. Obviously, she was a woman who knew a little something about trusting your instincts.

I said to myself, "Here's your moment, Lisa. What are you going to do?" By that point, I was all strapped into my bike, and it would have been so easy to stay there, but I told myself, "You've got to do this right now. Do it. Get off the bike, and walk over to her." Those were the scariest ten steps of my life. When I got to Andrea's bike, I said to her, "I want to congratulate you on *Dancing with the Stars*. What a brilliant move. I'm such a jerk for not doing it. I'm the biggest fool on earth for passing on it. I blew it, and I just wanted to say that, and congratulations." Then I walked back to my bike and got on. She was very gracious about it, and I was glad I had owned up to my mistake. I didn't expect anything to come of it—I just wanted to acknowledge my bad move and congratulate her on a job well done.

A few months later, I got a call from the people at *Dancing with the Stars*. They wanted to know if I was interested in doing season two of the show. This time I said, "I don't care what anyone says, I'm doing it." That phone call completely changed my life. I was still scared to death about dancing on national television, but I knew I had been given this opportunity for a reason, and I wasn't going to let it slip away a second time. I knew my passion for exercise had led me to this moment. If I hadn't been in that particular spinning class, I never would have had that life-changing conversation with Andrea Wong. And if I hadn't done so many years of aerobic exercises, I don't think I could have endured the grueling preparation for the show.

As an actress, you need to always look your best, which often can lead to self-destructive ways of staying slim and attractive. I know one of the reasons I haven't fallen prey to the many pitfalls of Hollywood—eating disorders, or drug or alcohol addiction, to name just two—is that exercise keeps me sane, and the process of staying fit gives me too much respect for my body to abuse it. Exercise makes me feel great, boosts my energy, and keeps me in good shape. It is my natural Prozac. But never in my wildest dreams could I have imagined that my love of working out would also open so many doors.

Exercise and fitness have been constants in my life since I was eight years old. I have no idea where my love of exercise came from, as neither of my parents was particularly athletic. My interest in exercise began with tennis. From age eight until I was seventeen, I played competitively in tournaments across the Pacific Northwest. But after almost ten years, the constant pounding ruined my knees, and I had to give it up. Instead of planting myself permanently on the living room sofa, I found a new pas-

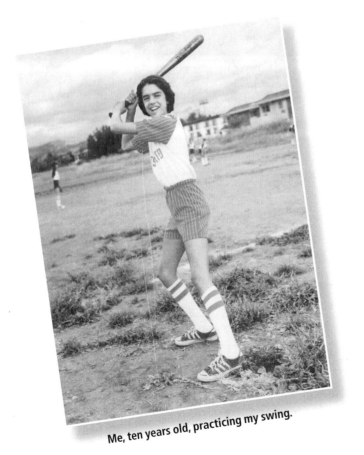

Me, ten years old, practicing my swing.

sion—Jazzercise. I loved it so much that I started teaching a class at a local racquet club when I was seventeen. Every morning at 6 A.M., I would set up my boom box and my cassette mix tapes of Kool and the Gang and K.C. and the Sunshine Band and lead my two or three early-bird students. The truth is I would have gotten up that early to Jazzercise even if I were all by myself; that's how good it made me feel. I loved the way it felt to move and stretch, and it cleared my head and pumped me up.

At eighteen, I went on to teach aerobics, and later after I moved to San Francisco, when I was twenty, I taught at a Richard Simmons studio. The studio was decorated like

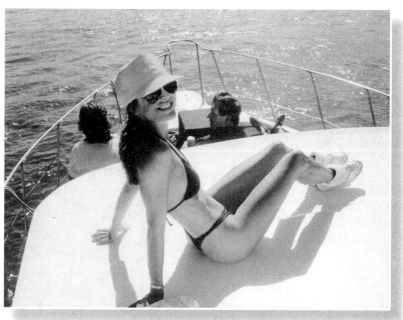

Rocking my Jazzercise body.

a disco, complete with red carpet, a disco ball, and dim lighting. I stood up on a stage, also red-carpeted (a sign of things to come?), and taught the class, still rocking my Kool and the Gang moves. Not only did I get to exercise to my heart's desire and be on stage at the same time, I was also helping others get in shape and feel good about themselves. I was in heaven.

I can clock my life by the kind of exercise I was doing during each phase. When I moved to Los Angeles, in my twenties, the first thing I did was sign up for Jane Fonda's aerobics classes. Since I was new in town, this was how I

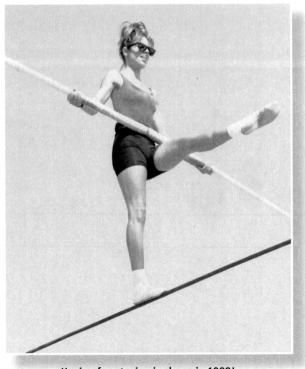

Having fun staying in shape in 1989!

met people. Some of my longest and strongest friendships have come from just showing up at the studio or gym, and I was always the first in line for the latest exercise trend.

In my thirties, during my *Melrose Place* days, I was devoted to Billy Blanks and his Tae Bo workout. Around that time, I also did Mari Winsor's Pilates, and Steve Ross's rock-and-roll yoga. Steve's class changed my life. I met so many people there—it was a social event, a pick-up place, really. I took that class for ten years straight, and I met some of my dearest friends there. The day I gave birth to my daughter Delilah, I took the class in the morning and gave birth later that night. (Throughout my two pregnancies, I always did something—Gurmukh prenatal yoga, walking, Pilates, anything that made me move and feel good. I know it helped me both physically and emotionally during labor.) Harry also took Steve's yoga class, and we had fun exercising together.

When I first heard of Sheila Kelley's S Factor classes, I knew I had to do it. I had recently had Delilah, and I felt unsexy, and dried up. I desperately needed to get my mojo back. I had read an article about her S (as in Strip) Factor in the *Los Angeles Times*, and a few days later, I saw her at a party; I made Harry go ask her about the classes (they had worked together on *L.A. Law*) because I was too embarrassed. At that time Sheila was teaching small groups of five to six women in her husband's office at her house. I started going to her house for lessons twice a week, and as with *Dancing with the Stars* later, the lessons opened a floodgate of emotions and loosened my inhibitions. The classes are a mixture of yoga, ballet, striptease, and pole dancing. Sheila teaches you how to do a striptease and work on the pole; the exercises require a lot of strength and force you to drop all inhibitions. You pick your own music and perform a sexy dance by yourself in front of the class, and you also learn how to do a lap dance! I did S Factor for four months straight, and then a few years later, after I had my daughter Amelia, I did it once a week for another four months in a private group at a friend's house in Malibu along with three of my close friends. It's a blast; you can wear lingerie and little short-shorts and stripper shoes that you buy on Hollywood Boulevard—anything you want—any kind of costume, any fantasy-related outfit or accessories you like. It really changed the way I feel about my body and my sexuality.

The most interesting thing to me about these sessions was observing how others reacted to the class. One of my friends is quite well known and felt self-conscious exhibiting herself in a big group at first. Ironically, she ended up loving it, and became so self-confident that she was soon a regular (and one of the best pupils) at the group classes! One woman was the most overtly sexual person I have ever met. She just oozed sex. Yet in the class she was very self-conscious and inhibited. She eventually loosened up and really took to it, but it took a while for that to happen. Contrary to the perception many people have of me, I tend to be very self-conscious about my body, especially at times in my life like right after giving birth, when I didn't feel so great about myself.

The S Factor taught me to appreciate my body in a way that exercise never had. As for Harry, let's just say he also learned to appreciate my body in a whole new way. It took a while for me to get up the nerve to dance for him (a whole year, to be exact), but let me tell you there is nothing like dancing for your man. It takes courage and confidence, but once you do it, it is incredibly empowering, and very hot. It is also an incredible workout. Working the stripper pole develops upper-body strength in your arms, chest, and abs. If there isn't an S Factor studio near you, pick up one of the DVDs and make your own party.

In my early forties, I started doing Barry's Boot Camp, which was featured on the television show *The Biggest Loser*. It's very intense and produces amazing results super-fast. The workout is an hour long, and includes thirty minutes of cardio on a treadmill and thirty minutes of strength training with free weights and military exercises. Their trademarked slogan is *The Best Workout in the World*. I found that it was a bit too intense for me—it made me feel like I was going to throw up—and made me look too muscular, so I stopped going to Boot Camp and mainly stuck to spinning and Pilates classes and a cardio circuit class. And, as I mentioned at the beginning of the chapter, spinning class led me to *Dancing with the Stars*, and again, committing to an exercise routine is about finding what works for you.

You would think my lifelong commitment to exercise would have made *Dancing with the Stars* a stroll in the park, but you would be wrong! The practice required to learn and perfect the routines and perform for the shows was both harder and more rewarding than anything I have ever done in my life. It also changed my body more than any of the exercise programs—I lost ten pounds and three inches from my waist. But the biggest impact was psychological. Though I wasn't conscious of it, I had years of bottled-up emotions that just flowed out of me when I danced. It was a daily roller coaster of emotions—from fear to frustration to exhilaration or despair, depending on how my practice or performance went. I cried all the time in rehearsal. I would become so frustrated when I couldn't master a move, and Louis Van Amstel, my dance partner, was tough (though, being such a perfectionist, I was even harder on myself).

I think everyone can relate to the experience of trying something new, and how hard it is to motivate yourself and keep going, especially when you feel like you'll never

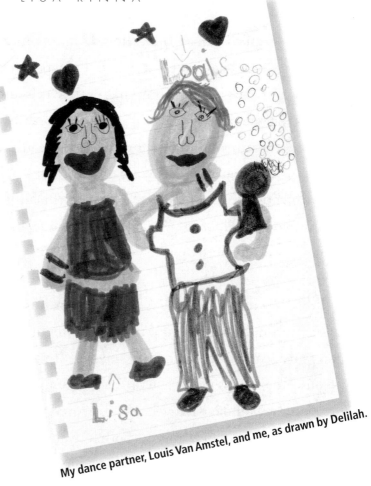

My dance partner, Louis Van Amstel, and me, as drawn by Delilah.

become good at it. But facing these fears and feelings gave me a greater sense of power and confidence than I had ever known. Most of all, it freed me—I let go of all my negative energy and fears of failure, and totally opened up my mind and body. And the best part was it wasn't a temporary fix; it was a permanent change in me and how I viewed the world.

All this from dancing? you ask. Absolutely. Suddenly,

amid the physical exhaustion, the self-punishment, the frustration, and the fear, it just gelled. I had been looking for a new challenge, something that both exhilarated me and pushed me to my breaking point; something that, when mastered, would make me feel that I could tackle anything. I encourage everyone to find their "Dancing with the Stars moment"; to try to do that thing you thought you couldn't do. The challenge alone will open a whole new world to you, if you just have the courage to try.

I didn't win *Dancing with the Stars*; for me it wasn't about winning, it was about putting myself out there and facing my fears, and challenging myself. It wasn't about the outcome, it was about the process. (Though don't get me wrong, I would have loved that mirrored ball trophy!) The lasting effects are many, both physical and emotional, but the biggest gift is the joy dancing still brings me. I put on music and my dance shoes and dance around the house, with my daughters or Harry, or sometimes just by myself. And every time, I get that same feeling of complete and utter bliss from doing something physical, graceful, and fun.

After going through the rigorous training of *DWTS*, I found myself really missing the discipline, and the physical and emotional effects of dancing. I'd learned that the older you get the more you've got to move it, and I was ready to keep moving it! So after I'd completed my stint on the show, I signed on to play Roxy Hart in *Chicago* on Broadway, which was another amazing and challenging experience—six months of nonstop dance! When that ended, in late August of 2007, I called Louis Van Amstel and told him, "Louis, we need to do a dance exercise class. I miss dancing, and I need it to keep my body in the shape it's been in for the past two and a half years!"

Louis and I rented a studio at Dove's Bodies in Studio City, where I had taken a cardio circuit class for the past eight years. We roughed out a routine for the class based on the *DWTS* routines and exercises, and then we called all my "mom" friends, and some of Louis's dancer friends, to come take the class. After the first class I knew we were on to something great. I knew it would be a gift for people who want to exercise and love to dance, and who want to try something new and fun and good for them. And so, cardio ballroom was born. We quickly outgrew the Studio City space and moved to a new location at Anisa's Dance Studio, in Sherman Oaks, right down the street from our Belle Gray store. We now have fourteen classes a week (!) and are looking to buy our own studio space. I absolutely believe that dancing is the best way to lose weight and get in shape because it doesn't feel like a fitness class. It's structured like an aerobics class, and no partner is needed. Louis leads the class, which is an hour long and totally high energy. It has basic salsa, cha-cha and jive steps, set to music by Mariah Carey, Cher, Gwen Stefani, and ABBA (which reminds me of my early Jazzercise classes!).

The response to the cardio ballroom class was so enthusiastic that Louis and I just produced a fourth cardio ballroom dance DVD set called *Lisa Rinna Dance Body Beautiful* with Warner Home video; DVD One is *Jive Jump Ballroom Bump*, DVD Two is *Ballroom Learn and Burn*, DVD Three is *Ballroom Body Blast* and DVD Four is called *Hip Hop Ballroom*. The dance routines work every part of your body and are really easy to follow. In addition to the instructive routines, we include sections on losing weight, getting fit, and dance basics. Some of the exercises are Rock-Out Dancer's Abs, Jive Jams for Tight Buns, Cardio Calf & Thigh Toner, and 555—five minutes, five times a week, to lose five pounds. I love it and never get tired of it. I can't stress enough that dancing is, by far, the best, fastest, and most fun way to get in the best shape of your life, and I'm so thrilled to be creating my own routine and sharing it with people, especially after spending so many years doing great programs taught by others.

Exercise continues to be a huge part of my daily life because I love it (especially dancing), and it's not a struggle for me to motivate myself to do it. I realize that not everyone feels the same way about exercising as I do, but I truly believe that once you start to do it and get into a routine that's right for you, you'll feel so much better (and look better too!). I mix it up to keep it interesting—Pilates, light weight training, yoga (which really changed my life by teaching me to be still and patient, as well as strong and flexible), kickboxing, dance, walking, running, or hiking (another new "find"). I also take a resistance class twice a week at the Tracy Anderson studio (Madonna and Gwyneth Paltrow train with Tracy, who is a former dancer. The goal of her program is to create long, lean dancer's muscles and tone, and there are big rubber bands suspended from the ceiling of her studio that we use during the class. It's a great cardio and toning workout—so fun and done to great music). These days, my exercise routine is probably more intense than most people would want to do, so I recommend finding what works for you and urge you to mix it up so you don't get bored. It doesn't matter how many hours or how many times a week you exercise, just do something. I try to exercise six days a week—that's what works for me.

Trust Me, It Works!

My eighty-six-year-old dad, Frank, works out six days a week. He goes to the gym and walks on the treadmill for twenty-five minutes and lifts light weights. I swear that's why he is still with us!

My Workout Routine

My philosophy is the more variety the better. Here's a sample week for me:

MONDAY: cardio ballroom class with Louis Van Amstel

TUESDAY: I train with a private trainer, Jeff DePeron (check out his website, huraathletics.com). We do ballet and tai chi movements with two-to-three-pound weights, with at least 15 to 25 reps per exercise. It helps me build long, lean muscles and keeps my bones strong to combat osteoporosis. I have low bone density, so weight-bearing exercises are a must for me, along with daily calcium supplements and small doses of sun for vitamin D.

WEDNESDAY: cardio ballroom

THURSDAY: Pilates, resistance class, or yoga. Or I'll run or walk on a treadmill and lift two-pound weights for one hour, or do some stretching and sit-ups on the big exercise ball and work out on the ab twister.

FRIDAY: cardio ballroom

SATURDAY: cardio ballroom or a spinning class (or both—I told you I love to exercise!).

SUNDAY: I take the day off. Even I need a rest!

✳

Don't get me wrong. As much as I love exercise, there are things about it I loathe. Ironically, given the "torture" of *Dancing with the Stars,* I don't like it when a trainer or teacher pushes me too hard. I feel like it's more about their proving how tough they are than it is about me. I also hate being sore after working out. A lot of people like this because it makes them feel that they've accomplished something—the whole "no-pain, no-gain" theory. But for me, if I feel sore, that means I've overdone it, and that isn't benefiting me or my body. (FYI, Epsom salt baths are great for treating soreness.) As I often say, extremes don't work for me. I would rather be moderate and consistent.

Also, as I've gotten older and have had to learn to juggle the responsibilities of career and family, I've realized that I need my exercise sessions to be very time-efficient. In my twenties, I would drive an hour each way to a studio to take an hour-and-a-half yoga class. Now I don't have that kind of time. I allow myself one hour, and choose classes that are easy to get to. I treat my workout as a mandatory appointment in my day. I also find that classes motivate me. I like working out with my friends and seeing the results they get. It inspires me, and I like that classes require another level of commitment to attend. The enthusiasm of the other attendees is also contagious—I get motivated with other people around me. Once I'm there, I push myself.

If you feel self-conscious exercising in front of people, or you don't have the time or money to go to classes, you can do everything in the privacy of your living room. There are great DVDs and videos for any and every exercise routine. There are also cable channels, like FitTV, that broadcast various workouts like Pilates, yoga, and body makeovers. And anyone, and I mean absolutely anyone, can dance. Just crank the music in your living room and let it all loose. The added bonus is that you can do each of these exercise programs in as little as twenty minutes a day, just by focusing on the area you want to improve. Make a promise to yourself that you will do something, anything, every day. It can be as little as a walk around the block—one step at a time. Hey, you can start moving your body when you're still sitting in a chair. The key is to *move*.

It's Not Just About Moving the Body

I'm not exaggerating when I say my love of exercise has made a significant impact on my life many times over. It has been my lifeline to sanity through many a rough time. It has also been an incredible social lifeline. When

I moved to Los Angeles, I met people while working out, whether it was aerobics class, yoga, or spinning. And of course, the Andrea Wong moment never would have happened if not for that Saturday morning spinning class. So my professional life has benefited from exercise as well. You never know who you'll meet when you walk into a gym!

I've always bonded with people through exercise, and Harry is no exception. When we first started dating, we would take long hikes to spend time together. One of our favorite things was climbing the Santa Monica steps. There are about a hundred steps and we would walk or jog up and down them until we were exhausted. (I do the same with my girlfriends. You can have much deeper conversations with people while on a walk or a hike than in a restaurant surrounded by tons of people.) Harry usually prefers to work out alone, doing weights at home, or taking day-long, off-the-trail hikes. He just recently hiked the Sierras by himself. He says hiking forces him to stay in the moment, because he focuses so hard on what he's doing that he can't think about other external things.

Harry and I also love to do physical activities with the girls. We bike ride, disco dance, jump on the trampoline, Roller-Blade, ice-skate, or bodysurf at the beach. Our family time is usually pretty active.

My Quick-Fix Workout

This routine is for when you need to get in shape fast, and it requires only a few pieces of equipment that you can easily store in your home. Doing these exercises, which concentrate on the upper body and core, every day for thirty days will lead to visible results—they are all you need to pull off that strapless dress or figure-hugging outfit.

I recommend that everyone have two- or three-pound weights at home. You should also have one of those rubber stretch bands with handles on both ends, and a big exercise ball. Keep them close by and do the following exercises while you are sitting at the computer or watching television.

Weights: the key to long, lean muscles and not bulking up is to use only two- or three-pound weights. I do three sets of 15 to 20 repetitions, and experiment with working the various muscles—pectoral muscles, biceps, and triceps. One of my favorite moves is to hold my arms straight out at shoulder level and lift them straight up over my head and down to my sides to work my entire upper body.

Band: work your pectorals, abs, and arms by holding each handle of the band and stretching it outward at chest level. Pull it out as far as you can, and then release it very slowly, controlling the motion. Do the same motion with the band behind your back at shoulder level.

Work the triceps and biceps by holding one end of the strap over your head with the other hand holding the strap between your shoulder blades. Extend the front arm straight up as far as you can, while pulling the back hand down your back.

Exercise ball: you can do sit-ups and curls, push-ups, and leg lifts with this one piece of equipment. Work your butt by draping your back over the ball with your hands and feet touching the floor. Slowly raise yourself off the ball and squeeze your butt muscles as many times as you can.

Sounds pretty easy, right? It is! And I know that once you start seeing the results you'll want to keep going and building on your routine. You don't have to spend hours in a gym or studio to move your body, and the equipment that you need to set up your own at-home fitness area is easy to stow under a bed and inexpensive to purchase. Trust me, every minute and every penny you spend on fitness is well worth the investment.

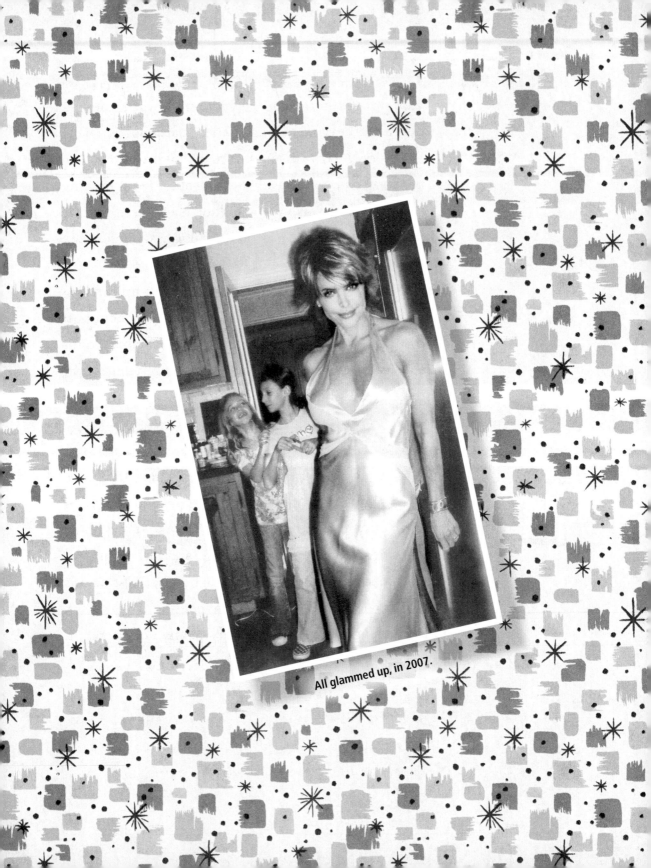

All glammed up, in 2007.

CHAPTER THREE

KICK-ASS BEAUTY

I've always been fascinated by the science of beauty. I am perpetually curious about every new cream, laser treatment, or miracle makeup that the dermatologist or beauty counter has to offer. Seriously, you name it, and I have tried it, sometimes with disastrous results. When I was pregnant with my first daughter, Delilah, I developed melasma, also known as the mask of pregnancy. I had brown spots all over my face. I had been getting facials for years, so I jumped at the chance to try a new glycolic peel from a facialist everyone was raving about, and I was optimistic that she could do something about my melasma.

I went to the facialist and she looked at my brown spots and said, "I can fix this. I can take this away completely. You'll never have another brown spot again." (Yeah, right.) She applied a combination of glycolic acid, salicylic acid, and a few other ingredients to my face. I remember thinking while she was doing it, "God, this stings." I'd never experienced that kind of burning on my face. Afterward, it's normal for your skin to appear red and a little raw for a few days (which is why you should always schedule a treatment at least two weeks before any special event). But the next day, instead of looking pink and splotchy, my face looked wind-burned and frostbitten, as if I had been in the Arctic. My skin was completely burned. It took me two years and many doctors to repair the damage. That it healed at all is a miracle. To this day, ten years later, I still have lingering brown spots that resemble a fading suntan, but at least I don't look like I was stranded on the tundra during a windstorm.

The story of my bad peel actually gets worse. While I was unknowingly having the worst peel of my life, the facialist started telling me about this great doctor in Beverly Hills who was injecting a miracle potion into people's faces—an all-natural, anti-wrinkle serum. "Injection parties" were all the rage in LA at the time. A group of women would get together at someone's house, and a doctor would make a house call and give them all shots of Botox or Restylane. The facialist told me the miracle potion was better than Botox or Restylane. You only had to do it once, and the results were permanent. I was chomping at the bit to try it, but the next day, after I saw what she had done to my skin, I figured I'd better take a pass on "Dr. Miracle Potion," at least for the time being. And thank God I did!

A few months later, a scandal was revealed—a doctor from Brazil was injecting Beverly Hills women with industrial, low-grade lubricant silicone called Articol. In plain English, that's the lubricant they use on automobile parts. The silicone injections had caused lumps, paralysis, and holes in the faces of some of the women. You guessed it—it was the same doctor my facialist from hell had recommended!

I thank heaven for dodging that bullet, and for the great lessons that experience taught me: always do your homework, and if something sounds too good to be true, it usually is. It also made me stop jumping at the chance to try the next big thing so quickly.

Was that near-miss the end of my quest for beauty? Not on your life. But I really do make sure to do my homework before I try anything new. In fact, I often joke that I could be a cosmetologist or dermatologist with all I've learned over the years through trial and error. In this chapter, I am going to tell you what works for me and people I know, and hopefully I will save you some time and money. I will share my makeup tricks and recommend creams, lotions, and facial treatments that can help you look younger. Some of these are what I call Pantry Face-lifts, which are potions you can whip up yourself with ingredients from your kitchen or pantry. I have solutions for breakouts, puffy eyes, sallow skin, whatever ails you. With all the new technology and science, plus a few old-fashioned home remedies, it's amazing what you can do with what God gave you. And the bottom line is if your face, hair, and skin aren't glowing, no one is going to notice your buff body or your killer outfit.

I'm going to focus on two ends of the spectrum—how to achieve a fabulous look for a special event, as well as tricks and tips you can use every day, even if you're just planning on running errands or doing your laundry. Let's be realistic—you're not going to wear fake eyelashes, hair extensions, and bright red lipstick every day, but you *can* begin and continue a skincare routine that makes your skin glow and your hair shine. Who doesn't want that?

Skin Boot Camp

I've had problem skin all of my life, so I've learned all the tricks to keep my skin looking healthy and glowing early on. I saw my first dermatologist when I was eleven years old, and I *still* get pimples. When I was in my twenties, I went to a hair salon that sold a line of all-natural skincare oils. I, of course, had to try them. Religiously,

I massaged the oil into my face twice a day. Two weeks later, I developed the worst acne of my life. I'm talking cystic acne, which causes big red pimples that you can't pop. I had about twenty of them on each cheek. Meanwhile, I was going on auditions for acting jobs. On one job I landed, the makeup artist tried to cover the acne with makeup, which of course only made it worse. At the time, it was the most traumatic experience of my life. I was twenty-seven years old, at a critical point in my career, and I looked like a freak.

My dermatologist put me on Accutane, which completely dries you up like a prune. I already felt like I was ready to jump off a roof, thanks to my flawed skin, but the side effects of the medication put me over the edge. To make matters worse, my doctor told me it would take three months for the medicine to kick in and deliver results, and my skin was going to get worse before it got better. It took an entire year to get my acne under control. At the time, I was in a bad relationship, which didn't help my state of mind. I now see it was related—psychosomatic. I was miserable inside and out. That's another factor related to your skin: the worse you feel inside, the worse your skin will look. Unfortunately, I don't have the antidote for that, but I can offer the dos and don'ts that will handle the rest.

If you have followed my diet plan and have begun eating the Fab Foods, you are already on your way to having healthy, beautiful skin. I eat these foods because they are the ultimate multitaskers. They not only help me lose weight and build muscle tone, but they also work at the cellular level, nourishing and hydrating my skin, and plumping it up so wrinkles disappear. In addition, they are reported to contain anti-aging properties. So think of eating the Fab Foods as priming the canvas before you create your masterpiece.

First, you need to whip your skin into shape. Have a professional facial, or give yourself an exfoliating facial. It's a big waste of time and money to pile new products on dead skin. You want to slough off all of the old lackluster skin layer so you are working with a clean slate. This would be a great time to visit a cosmetologist or dermatologist to find what your skin needs. Whether you are combating wrinkles, acne, or just a dull skin tone, they can recommend the right products. You can also ask an expert, be it a cosmetologist, makeup artist, or dermatologist, what the various ingredients in moisturizers do, and what makeup is best for your skin type and tone. It can be incredibly confusing, not to mention irritating (literally), to figure out the difference between hydraluronic, salicylic, and glycolic acids, as they all do very different things, and the price variations are tremendous, so it's good to seek an expert opinion. Then, once you know what your skin needs, you can do research on the Internet and find out which products fit your price range. Here's a little secret: I know celebrities who swear by a certain $250 face cream. I've tried it and wasn't all that impressed. Then a makeup artist recommended a face lotion, GlyDerm Lotion Lite, with comparable ingredients, and it knocked my socks off. The best part? It costs only $22. Again, find what works for your skin type.

Be sure to shop around by calling local salons and explaining that you have a special event coming up, and ask if they have any packages or promotions, such as facials, spray tans, exfoliating, or waxing. Usually, they will try to accommodate you if they think you might become a regular client.

I have learned over the years to listen to my skin. I can feel when it is dry, oily, or dull-looking and react accordingly. I apply masks once or twice a week. There are so many to choose from, I like to mix it up and do a cleansing one night, a lifting mask another, an oxygen mask a different night—you get the picture. Cleansers are also a key part of my beauty routine because I have oily, blemish-prone skin. And anti-aging creams and lotions are a must! I started using them a few years ago and I apply them religiously. I vary the products and routines, depending on how my skin looks and feels, and where I am climate-wise—New York, Los Angeles, or other parts of the country. But usually less is more!

Beyond Boot Camp

After you've had a facial and figured out what sort of products to apply, you might want to consider fillers such as Botox, Restylane, or Juvéderm, if your budget permits and you're not queasy about needles. These give immediate results and last for about six months. Every four months or so, I get Botox to fill in my crow's-feet and the furrows in my brow, and Restylane for my smile lines. When I was doing *Soaptalk*, we did a segment where my cohost and I were to get Botox injections on air. I chose to do mine off-air, but I might as well have done it live, because the next day my face was completely frozen. I couldn't move my forehead or my eyebrows for three months! It was obvious what I'd done, and everyone laughed (okay, not everyone—Harry just shook his head). I hated the feeling of being

frozen, but I laughed along too, and since that experience, I'm very careful about not getting "frozen face."
After all, as an actress, you need to be able to move your
face to show expression. If you ever have too much filler
put in at once, back off for a while. The plumpness will
go down after a few months. Just don't do anything that
is permanent!

THE LIPS

Admit it—you were dying to get to this part! The one
thing people comment on more than my hair is my lips.
I've never addressed the speculation publicly before because I felt it was my business, and no one else's. I'm generally with Madonna, who says, "I'm not against plastic
surgery. I'm just against talking about it." But since I'm
baring everything else in this book, I figure I have to come
clean about "the lips," and address the pink elephant in
the room. Okay, here goes. . . .

When I was in my twenties, my friend and I watched
the movie *Beaches*. We couldn't get over Barbara Her-
shey's lips. We thought they were the coolest things we
had ever seen (crazy, I know!). Beauty fanatic that I am,
I thought I had found the key to being gorgeous—lips.
Boy, was I insecure at the time. I had always had a full
bottom lip but my upper lip was, to me, too thin and out

of proportion compared to my bottom lip. So my friend and I made appointments with a Beverly Hills doctor and we had collagen injected into our upper lips. The result was cool—painful, but I loved it. I felt sexy, pretty, exotic, and a little bit naughty. The only problem was the collagen injections lasted only about three months.

Then I got a brilliant idea. I heard that a lot of people were getting silicone injections, which offered permanent results (I know; most logical people would see a big red flag there, but not me, Little Miss Gullible.) It sounded like the answer to my prayers. So I found a doctor in Beverly Hills. (Don't worry, while this was over two decades ago, the silicone my doctor used was hospital-grade purified silicone—not like the stuff the Brazilian doctor was using.) The series of four treatments was long and excruciatingly painful because the doctor had to inject little beads of silicone into my lips drop by drop. My girlfriend and I would go together, and we'd squeeze each other's hands during the injections because the pain was so bad. Afterward, we would go to the Hamburger Hamlet, which was below the doctor's office, and giggle and put ice on our lips. Sounds insane, doesn't it? Ah, youth!

It seemed completely worth it—I loved my plump lips, and they were mine forever. That is, until the scar tissue developed. What happens is, over time, the silicone hardens and scar tissue starts to form (or *deform* might be a better word) underneath the lips, and little bulges erupt from the scar tissue. Gross, I know. People constantly speculate about my lips, saying they have gone up and down in size over the years. Recently, someone even said that I admitted on *The Howard Stern Show* that I had inflatable lip implants, which I could inflate and deflate at will. Not true!

Another source said I had spent $150,000 on my lips. If I did, they had better be lined with gold! In truth, the only thing I've done in the twenty years since I got the silicone injections is try to take them down a little. To do this, the doctor slowly injects cortisone into my lips to soften the hardened silicone. This makes the lips look slightly smaller and softer. Short of surgery, there is no way to completely get rid of the scar tissue, and I know people who have had surgery, which entails cutting the lips open and taking out the silicone and scar tissue. It doesn't work and permanently mutilates you. No thanks! The truth is, I still love my lips. They are part of me, and they have become what I am known for, for better or worse. In any case, they're permanent, so I could either live my life with regret or embrace my choice. Which do you think is the better way to live? I've always been impetuous and impatient—I still am—but I wouldn't change a thing except my insecurity (well, maybe I would also skip that glycolic peel I got when I was pregnant).

My favorite treatments for looking young and fresh, courtesy of Kate Somerville Skin Care:

- The Genesis laser treatment from Kate Somerville is amazing for stimulating collagen.
- The Derma Quench Hydrating Facial, also from Kate Somerville, is an oxygen and hyaluronic acid treatment that was created for skin cancer patients. This treatment is one of my all-time favorites. It heals your skin right before your eyes, and plumps it up, evens out skin tone, and repairs the texture.
- Twice a year, I get a Cosmelon facial peel. It lightens brown spots like nothing else!
- Every month, I get the Blue Light/Red Light treatment at Kate Somerville, for breakouts. It kills bacteria, heals the skin, and stops further breakouts. Because I've always had problem skin, I get these treatments religiously. These may not be right for your skin, and you may find other treatments more beneficial. The point is to figure out what works for you and to get into a routine. But always remember to do your homework and don't let anyone talk you into something you don't feel comfortable with. I developed my beauty routine over years of trial and error, research, and seeking recommendations.

All of it, mistakes and all, has made me who I am today. And I hope that by sharing my story I've helped others who might be tempted to try any sort of procedure to know that you need to be very careful about permanently changing your face, whether you're considering a nose job, chin or cheek implants, anything. I always say your goal should be to look like you, just better or younger. You have to be true to the face and genes you have—what Mother Nature gave you. Again, if a procedure or treatment sounds too good to be true, it probably is. As you'll see below, there are so many things you can do with makeup and skin potions that are not irreversible. Unless you are one hundred percent sure you want to have cosmetic surgery, just enjoy and work with what you've got.

Back to Basics: My Favorite Home Remedies

If you don't have the time, money, or interest in seeking skin advice from a professional, or in purchasing sometimes costly products, here are some of my favorite home remedies. These are my Pantry Face-lifts, the do-it-yourself treatments I have picked up over the years from cosmetologists, friends, and magazines. Not only do they work for me, but they are also easy and inexpensive to make.

- **To lighten age spots**, mix the juice of 1 lemon, 1 lime, 2 tablespoons of honey, and 2 ounces of plain yogurt together in a bowl. Yogurt contains a natural bleaching property (and it's one of the Fab Foods!). Rub the mixture into each spot, including sun-damaged cleavage. Do this several times before you need to attend a big event, and your skin will look even and gorgeous.

- **To make my absolute favorite face tightener and pore minimizer**, beat 1 egg white to a froth. Apply the foamy liquid to your entire face, focusing on problem areas around the jaw, eyes, and forehead. Let it dry completely (about ten minutes), then gently rinse and pat dry.

- **To combat under-eye bags**—there are many tried-and-true remedies for this problem—try placing cucumber slices, raw potato slices, moistened tea bags, or chilled spoons over each eye. Leave them on for ten minutes or so, then check your results. Repeat until bags disappear.

- **To reduce puffiness around the eyes:** Preparation H is an old tried-and-true prescription for shrinking eye puffiness. It works, but some people find the ointment greasy and/or are put off by its smell (or just the idea of it). I am one of those people. Someone told me to try Tucks pads, and guess what? They work just as well as Preparation H and are odor- and grease-free. You can use them on your neck, jaw line, or forehead—any place that needs quick tightening.

- **To make a fantastic moisturizing mask**, mash up an avocado and apply it to your face. You'll look scary while it's on, but after removing it with warm water you'll see that it works.

- **To make my excellent exfoliator**, mix a few table-spoons of sugar with a few tablespoons of olive oil or water, if you have acne-prone skin. Gently massage the mixture all over your face. Rinse with warm water and pat dry.

- **To make a gentle exfoliator**, make a paste of baking soda and water and rub the mixture all over your skin. Rinse thoroughly with warm water and pat dry.

- **To make a clay mask**—which is great for pulling tox-ins out of your skin—some facialists use (I kid you not) 100 percent clay kitty litter. (I told you I'd try anything!) It contains the same ingredients that are in the expensive clay masks. Make a paste of the clay by mixing it with water, and apply to your skin. Let it sit until it hardens, and then rinse with warm water and pat dry.

- **To make your own collagen booster**, mash 1 cooked carrot with 1 avocado, then add ½ cup heavy cream and blend. Apply the cream to your face and neck and leave it on for fifteen minutes. Then rinse with cool water. The beta-carotene in the carrot, the vitamin E in the avocado, and the calcium in the heavy cream combine to boost collagen levels, lighten age spots, and improve overall skin tone. Do this once a week for a month and your face will glow.

- **To use oils to your advantage:** coconut oil is a miracle moisturizer on dry hair, nails, feet, you name it. Olive oil is a legendary Mediterranean beauty secret for supple, soft skin—rub it on your skin, your feet, and your nails. To condition and repair damaged hair, combine $^1/_2$ cup of olive oil and 2 to 3 sprigs of fresh rosemary and let it sit overnight. The next day, remove the rosemary, and massage the oil into your hair; let it soak in for ten to fifteen minutes, and rinse with warm water. Then shampoo to get rid of the oil residue. Sesame oil is another great all-over body moisturizer. Neutrogena makes a body oil that is super light and smells heavenly; apply it to damp skin after you shower for a smooth, subtle sheen that also accentuates muscle tone and enhances a tan. Right before I step onto the red carpet, I like to rub a little lavender oil on my arms and legs. It smells great, and it makes my skin soft and silky.

- **To make a lip exfoliator**—you should try to exfoliate your lips once a week to get rid of dead skin and plump them up—mix a paste of honey and sugar and rub the mixture on your lips. Then use a tooth-brush to slough off the dead skin.

- **To make an instant lip plumper**, simply rub cinnamon on your lips. It's that easy.
- **To make my ultra hand moisturizer**, blend 1 egg yolk, 1 tablespoon of honey, 2 tablespoons of extra-virgin olive oil, 1 tablespoon of sugar, and 2 drops of lemon essential oil. Use it every time you wash your hands and your hands will be silky smooth in no time.

You may have realized that a lot of the above products are used for getting rid of dead skin and moisturizing. *I cannot stress enough the importance of moisturizing*, especially your hands! I moisturize my hands every night. I like to double the impact by wearing sleep gloves to bed once a week to keep the cream on my hands and off my sheets. I love Aquaphor, which is inexpensive and can be found in any drugstore. I also really like Palmer's Cocoa Butter Formula Jar, which I use on feet, knees, and elbows. And I *always* apply sunscreen before I walk out the door.

If you are not the weekly manicure type, and many of us aren't (or can't be), keep your routine simple. Keep your fingernails and toenails clipped and your skin smooth and callus-free. You don't need a French manicure to look polished, but you shouldn't be walking around with rough-looking skin and ragged, chipped nails.

Pamper your hands once a week by filing and clipping your nails, coating them in hand lotion or Vaseline, and then wearing moisturizing gloves to bed. You can make this a relaxing ritual by doing it while you are watching television during a night in. Use aromatherapy or essentials oils to relax or lift your mood. Apply a bold color to your toenails to jazz them up. Have fun while you groom!

And please be diligent about exfoliating and moisturizing your feet. For dry, cracked feet, once a week slather them with moisturizer and then cover them with socks or plastic-lined booties before bed. You can also purchase a foot spa for as little as $25; not only is it soothing to use, but it will soften your rough spots and make it easier to groom your toenails.

A non-negotiable beauty routine for every woman is wearing sunblock. I wear sunscreen every day. Your daily moisturizer must have an SPF of at least 30, preferably higher. Neutrogena makes a very light, non-greasy lotion with an SPF of 30 or 45 that I like, and I'll also use either Dr. Lancer's SPF 50 or Kate Somerville Protect SPF 30 on my face. They are specially formulated for the face so they are not too heavy or greasy. Never leave home without it! The brown spots will come right back if you don't wear sunscreen every day.

The Best Skin Quick Fix

A great trick that I learned from the professional dancers on *DWTS* is that a tan makes you look thinner. It also makes you feel healthier—an added bonus. So a fabulous faux tan is my favorite quick fix. Unless you've been living in a cave, you know that the worst thing for your skin is sun. But let's be honest—everyone looks better with a tan. *Everyone.* It used to be that your only choices for a fake tan were the lotions that turned you orange, not bronze, and invariably left streaks and blotches of color. *So* unattractive. But hallelujah, technology came to the rescue, and now you can sport a bronze glow all year round. Here is my routine:

I begin by applying a moisturizing self-tanning cream after my shower to subtly build a base. I rub a big gob between my palms and spread it evenly all over, the way you do suntan lotion, making sure not to miss spots. Then I spray a bronzing mist all over (most come in light, medium, and dark so you can work your way up to the shade you want). This stuff is the best. Because it sprays on as a thin mist, there are no streaks or blotches. It doesn't stain clothes or the palms of your hands, and you can find brands that cost as little as $10. Products I like are Neutrogena's Sunless sprays and lotions and MAC's Bronze

Glitter Self-Tanner. I use Tan Towels swipe-on cloths to add quick, subtle color to my face, chest, and arms; it's especially good for combating winter pallor. Finally, I get a professional spray tan at a tanning salon. With a nice base, the spray tan blends with your skin tone and looks more genuine. (You can also ask the tanning person to "sculpt" parts of your body. By strategically applying darker tanner on biceps or inner thighs, or even on your abs, you can make them look more toned and sculpted.)

Now that you're "tan," remember to massage a big chunk of cocoa butter or solid coconut oil into your skin after you take a shower. (You can find good-quality brands of cocoa butter and solid coconut oil at health food stores.) If I'm going out for a special occasion, I apply the self-tanner as usual, and then rub sesame or almond oil (Clarins body oil is also yummy, and has a bonus use: applied with cocoa butter, this oil prevented me from getting stretch marks while I was pregnant) all over my body for a golden-goddess vibe. (I also love Epicuren Orange Blossom, and Lavender body cream, Origins Volcanic Mud Mask, and Nivea Moisturizer for the body. I told you, I love beauty products!)

Quick-Fix Mini-tip!

Remember what your mother taught you: nothing beats a great smile. If your teeth could use a bit of polish, there are a plethora of over-the-counter whitening products as well as whitening trays and laser treatments you can get from your dentist. Because your smile is so important, you might want to consider cosmetic procedures if whitening doesn't do the trick. Ask your dentist about bonding, veneers, and laminates. The costs vary, but it is one of those investments that lasts a lifetime and can transform your face more than you can even imagine. And your choice of toothpaste matters too—my favorite is Arm & Hammer's baking soda and peroxide toothpaste. It keeps my teeth looking really white.

Makeup Magic

Now that you have the perfect canvas, let's focus on the painting. The best way to nail your perfect look is to go to any department store cosmetician and describe what you're looking for and enlist her help. Bring photos of your favorite model or celebrity, and point out what you like about their look. While you're there, ask the cosmetician to suggest products to use for special occasions, in addition to the ones you'll use for your everyday look. Have her apply both looks; if you're not happy with them, say so and keep experimenting. Make it fun—pretend you are a celebrity and you are auditioning this person to be your personal makeup artist. Ask for her professional opinion on various products—cleansers, moisturizers, foundation. Which does she like and why? Which would she recommend for you? Sample the makeup like a kid in a candy store with no obligation to buy, and if the salesperson is pushy, try somewhere else. Enjoy your free makeup lesson, and if you want additional tips, you can also go online at home and do some research. It's amazing how much you can learn online from the customer reviews of products alone. Sephora.com and beauty.com are two sites I highly recommend. The Editor's Picks on allure.com are also terrific.

MY BEAUTY ROUTINE

These are some of the products I use every day: for my lips, I go very minimal: MAC Prrr lip gloss, and Chapstick (the original—I can't live without it!). I use Nars Ginger Concealer under my eyes and to even out any splotches. For a little more polish, I use Nars Barbarella lipstick, Nars Orgasm blush, Bobby Brown Oil-Free Even Finish

Cream Base, and Chanel Bronzer Liquid Shimmer. I also like Bobbi Brown pressed powder in Sunny Beige and Guerlain Terracotta Bronzing Powder #2. And I love my Shu Uemura eyelash curler.

My Personal Makeup Quick Fix

My favorite quick fix for getting gorgeous in a second is false eyelashes. I don't use any particularly fancy brand of lashes; the strips that you can buy at the drugstore work just fine. They make your eyes look gigantic, and are so glamorous. I recommend trimming a little off the outer edge before applying, which will give you a cool cat-eye look.

Hair: Mane Inspiration

I like short hair. It works for me, and I never change it. I think if you have a few staples—a good husband, the perfect little black (or red or fuchsia) dress, and a great haircut, you should hang on to them for dear life, and ignore the urge to "try something new." Your hairstyle makes or breaks your look and defines your own personal style. Think about women who have a signature hairstyle—

Goldie Hawn, Jane Fonda, Jennifer Aniston, Farrah Fawcett. It's hard to imagine them without picturing their hair; it is so integral to their persona. The trick is finding out what hairstyle and color are most flattering to you, and sticking with them. It took me years, but when I finally found the perfect stylist, I held on for dear life. I've had this same haircut for almost two decades.

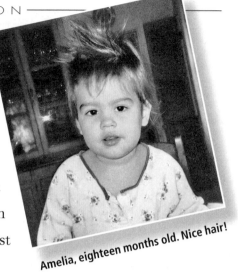

Amelia, eighteen months old. Nice hair!

My 1992 hairstyle inspiration came from a girl in my acting class, who had the cutest haircut. I went to her stylist and got the same haircut she had. I had auditioned for *Days of Our Lives* a few days before my salon appointment, and hadn't yet gotten the part. But when I went to the callback with my new haircut, I got the part. I know, without a doubt, that my hair is the reason I got the part. Without consciously planning it, I had given myself a signature look that set me apart from everyone else and gave me a sassy confidence I didn't have before. I had also recently begun seeing Harry at that time, and he was always urging me not to cut my hair and to grow my hair longer. I gave in once, after I gave birth to my daughter Delilah, and I hated it.

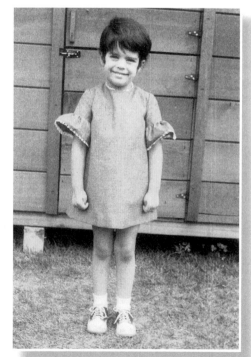

Me, age three and a half, showing off my new haircut in front of my playhouse.

It made my face look too long and drawn-out. I think you are either a long-haired girl or a short-haired girl. Sure, over the years, I've experimented with the cut and color a little bit, but never so much that I lose this look. Although there was one cut, right before I got the role on *Melrose Place*, that was a bit drastic. My hair was fairly long (for me), and I was dying to do something different. I had been away at an acting workshop in Vermont, and the first place I went when I got back to Los Angeles was to my hair stylist Jonathan Antin. I had him cut my hair very short, into a pixie cut—very Mia Farrow. I loved it. When I got home, I walked into Harry's office. He took one look at me, and without a word, he buried his head in his hands. He wouldn't have sex with me for three months! (I swear!) He never said anything; he just acted distant and a little strange. Finally, after it had grown out a bit, he came back around, but it was a very long three months. I will never cut my hair that short again!

Bottom line: Your hair is one of the first things people notice about you, coming and going. The great thing about hair is it grows back and, nowadays, with extensions and wigs, you can change it up in a snap. I did experiment with my hair while doing *Dancing with the Stars*—it was fun to change my hair so it looked appropriate for the dance and I learned that I love having my hair slicked back in a bun. But you should try to figure out what works for you, develop a signature style, and then fight the desire to mess with a good thing!

Hair Color and Style
Splurging vs. Saving

This is one area where you don't want to skimp. Find the best hairstylist and the best colorist (this is rarely the same person, and you want someone who specializes in one or the other). You might want to give them a trial run for a couple of months before a big event in case it doesn't work out. Think of picking a top-notch stylist and colorist as making a long-term investment. I know it can be expensive, but it's worth it. If it really looks that fabulous, find a way to cut corners somewhere else. I'm just saying. . . . Certain things are important, right?

After you find the right cut, the next step is color. Thankfully the beauty rules have changed, and you no longer have to worry about matching your skin tone and eye color to your hair color (remember when the beauty magazines would insist that if you have dark skin and eyes, you must have dark hair?). Now, there are so many different techniques and products available that a good colorist can make any shade flatter your face.

Before you start playing with color, first do your research. There are websites on which you can upload a photo of yourself and superimpose different hairstyles and colors onto your face to see if they complement your skin tone and hair texture. (There are similar sites for "trying on" clothes; isn't technology amazing?) While it's possible to make adjustments to your hair color after it's been dyed, it's always best to get it right on the first try. Spare your hair the extra chemicals!

MY EVERY DAY HAIR ROUTINE

Because I work out six days a week, I have to be careful not to dry out my hair through constant shampooing. My salvation is a product called Wen made by Chaz Dean. Wen is a cleansing conditioner that you use as a shampoo, and it keeps my hair healthy and undamaged. I alternate between using Wen three days a week, and Kerastase shampoo and conditioner the other four. I also love Kerastase Nutritive Serum Nutri-Sculpt, a shine enhancer. And I use Paul Mitchell mousse, Tea Tree Styling Wax, Magic Move Pomade, Kerastase hairspray, and L'Oréal Elnett hairspray, which is expensive but it lasts a long time. (I'm a big believer in switching things up; I never use the same product two days in a row.) For styling, I just blow-dry my hair with mousse and a round brush, put a little pomade in it, and I'm good to go. My cut is very wash-and-go and low maintenance, which suits me perfectly.

> ## Opposite of Quick Fix: Getting Red-Carpet Ready
>
> Getting red-carpet ready with Team Rinna requires the help of Faye Woods (hair), Adam Christopher (makeup), and Jen Rade (stylist), and takes two hours, soup to nuts. That's right. *Two hours.*

My Three-Week-Long Red-Carpet Prep Routine

Here's a quick breakdown of what I do to get red-carpet ready. I already told you it takes two hours of hair, makeup, and styling on the day of the event, but that's just the tip of the iceberg! And in addition to the below list, I watch what I eat and I rev up my workouts.

Three weeks before: I get my hair trimmed, color the base, and get highlights.

Two weeks before: I do an at-home facial treatment for fifteen minutes using Bliss's Steep Clean, then I apply

Origins Clear Improvement Mud Mask for thirty minutes. I finish with Bliss Spa's Triple Oxygen Face Mask.

One week before: I deep-condition my hair, and get a Genesis laser treatment and a Derma Quench facial from Kate Somerville, for really fresh, glowing skin.

Two days before: I get a spray tan from Portofino Sun. They mix this really beautiful color that looks so healthy and glowing. I also get a manicure and pedicure, and I try to get eight hours of sleep for the next couple of nights.

Voila! I'm ready for the professionals to take over on the day of the big event.

I know my routine might sound rigorous, but it all boils down to a few key elements that you can use to get gorgeous before any big event—taking extra care to make sure your hair and skin look great, and giving yourself enough time to do so. Yes, makeup can help glam you up on the big day, but once you get the invitation, you should pull out your calendar and mark off when you're going to begin your beauty prep, approximately three weeks before the actual event.

And now that we've laid the foundation for your new look, you're ready for some window dressing. . . .

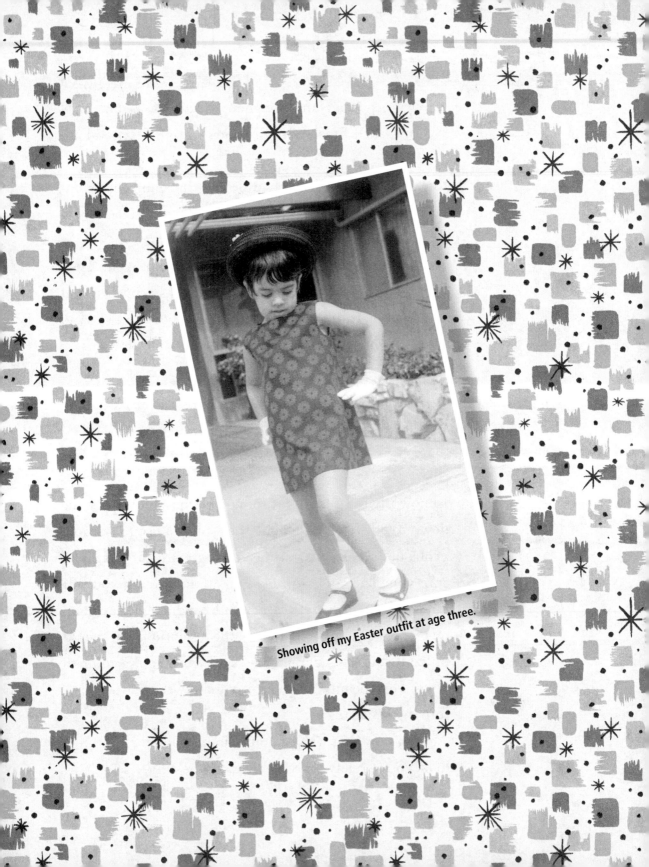

Showing off my Easter outfit at age three.

CHAPTER FOUR

A PASSION FOR FASHION

I grew up in Medford, Oregon, where there was not one cool store to shop in. There wasn't even a mall in town when I moved there in 1970. It was the most boring place on the planet, as far as I was concerned. My family had relocated to Medford from sunny Newport Beach, California, when I was seven, and you can't imagine two more different worlds. In Newport Beach, the style was Florence Eisenman prints and mini-Izod dresses, which my mother hemmed right up to my crotch. It was a whole different story in Medford. The uniform of choice in my new home was wide-leg Chemin de Fer jeans and rocker tees—hardly the stuff of *Vogue* magazine. Everyone was all-American looking: light-haired and fair-skinned, and the cool haircut to have was the mullet.

When I was in my teens, my mom noticed my interest in fashion and got me a subscription to *Seventeen* maga-

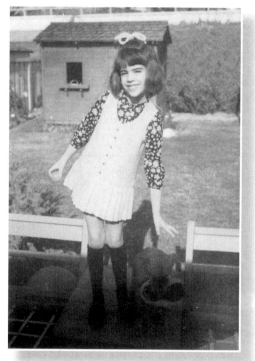

Already a fashionista at age six.

zine, and later *Glamour* and *Vogue*. I loved the models on the pages of these glossies—it was the era of Kelly Emberg, Christie Brinkley, and Kim Alexis. They became my idols, and fashion was an escape from my mundane life. To earn money to buy clothes, I took a job as a salesclerk at Lerner's, a discount department store, when I was fifteen. I'd save the money until my family and I would make one of our semi-annual trips to San Francisco to visit my grandmother, and this is where I would shop. I'd head to I. Magnin, Joseph Magnin, and Macy's, which were so much cooler and more up to date with the trends than Lerner's, and I'd buy the clothes I had seen in the magazines—stylish, fashion-forward pieces; things you couldn't find in the stores in Oregon—with the money I saved up from my Lerner's job. (In retrospect, that should have been a red flag.) The summer of my freshman year, I took my hard-earned money from Lerner's and bought my first pair of straight-leg jeans and Candies shoes, and the *pièce de résistance*: a burgundy cashmere sweater dress with buttons down the entire back of the dress, which I intended to pair with new brown suede pumps. I thought I was super-groovy cool!

The first day of school, I wore the burgundy sweater dress and the brown pumps, which I could barely walk in. Not only were my peers not blown away by my fashion savvy, they teased me mercilessly; I was totally ridiculed. To them, I didn't look urban and chic but, instead, out of place, foreign, even scary. I came home in tears, and I never wore that outfit again (though I kept the sweater dress until I was in my twenties). Humiliating as that experience was, it did nothing to kill my love of fashion. I thought, okay, these people aren't ready for that. And I learned two important lessons—first, life is going to be cruel, and second, I was different from everyone else, and I had to accept and embrace that fact or get a mullet haircut to blend in. "Not."

With my dark hair and skin, I didn't look like anyone else in my school, and dealing with the challenge of being different from my peers has pretty much made me who I am. (There were no African American or Asian students at my school at the time.) My passion for fashion has been both a factor that sets me apart and a coping mechanism. I believe that being fashionable is not about money, it's about tapping into your passion, working with what you have, and staying true to who you are. I have always loved vintage shops and flea markets, where you can find great stuff—I found my favorite pair of cowboy boots at the Rose Bowl flea market! You really don't have to spend a lot to have great fashion.

I feel that fashion empowers me. It is the ultimate game of dress-up, and it is a creative outlet, a way to make myself feel sensual, sexual, pretty, glamorous, tomboyish, or athletic—through clothes I can take on any person or mood I choose. Angie Dickinson famously said, "I dress for women, but I undress for men." While I definitely undress for my husband, I dress for myself. When I feel great about myself, it affects the way everyone around me responds, because there is no greater combination than confidence and a great outfit. Even if I wasn't in the public eye, I would look exactly like I do. My style is just who I am.

Being interested in fashion is not about vanity, and it

doesn't mean that you're superficial or shallow. I think fashion is great, and I love clothes. If I allowed myself to trivialize this or any of the things that are important to me, I would never accomplish anything. Hey, I was able to turn my passion into a multimillion-dollar business!

I've said I can clock my life through the exercise program I was doing at the time, and the same is true with my fashion choices. The evolution of my personal style coincides with very specific periods in my life. When I was in my twenties and working on *Days of Our Lives*, people started taking notice of what I wore as photos of me appeared in the daytime soap opera magazines. But I hadn't yet crossed over to the "big time," the national magazines. Then in 1992, I was invited to the Carousel Ball, Nancy Davis's biannual charity fund-raiser, and I knew I wanted to wear something fabulous. I found *the dress*—it was white with a gold belt looped through the waist, and it was all open on one side. The designer was Tom Ford for Gucci; he wasn't a big name then but I sensed he would be. The dress cost $1,300, which I didn't have, but my instincts told me to go for it, so I maxed out my credit card. That dress changed everything for me. The next week photos of me in that white dress ran in every national magazine on the newsstands. Always eager to outdo myself, for the next Carousel Ball in 1994, I wore a black Versace dress with tiny cutouts on the side. Harry and I were there together as a couple this time around. Once again, the media took notice and the photos led to more exposure.

I sensed the power of style back in high school, when I wore that burgundy sweater dress. But now people, instead of making fun of me, were saying, "Wow, you look great! Where did you get that? How did you put it together?" People were paying attention to me because of what I wore, and somewhere in the back of my mind, the idea for my clothing boutiques was born. I was indulging

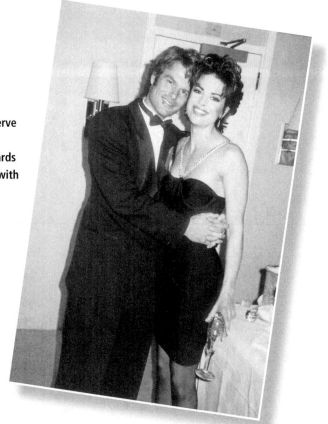

Glammed up in Herve Leger at the Soap Opera Digest Awards in 1992. I hosted with Kelsey Grammar.

my passion for fashion *and* getting lots of attention and approval, so why not make a business out of it? Though I wouldn't open the first Belle Gray store until almost a decade later, the seed was definitely planted.

Sixteen years ago, the "who are you wearing?" red-carpet coverage that is so prevalent today did not exist. (That started only about twelve years ago, with the rise of Joan and Melissa Rivers.) Since being noticed for my clothes was a new thing, and I love to push the boundaries, this was an awesome time for me. In the late nineties, celebrities like Toni Braxton, Carmen Electra, Heather Locklear, and Jennifer Lopez were wearing daring, risqué designs, especially at the edgier music awards shows. They were the perfect opportunity to play extreme dress-up, so in 1997 (during my *Melrose Place* stint), when I was a presenter at the American Music Awards, I teased my hair really wild—too wild—and wore a yellow gown cut all the way up to my armpit, with only a tiny little string holding it together at the hip. It was really out there, and I loved it. My feeling is if it scares you a little, it's probably good. Why not go for it?

Years later, when I was on *Dancing with the Stars*, Louis Van Amstel and I designed our own dance outfits. In the beginning Louis did most of the clothes, because he knew the dances and the best styles and colors for them. Slowly I started getting more involved in picking the clothes (especially when it came to choosing the colors, because I know which colors work for me and my coloring and which don't). Louis designed the dresses for the first two dances. The first was a leopard-print number and totally out of the box for a waltz. The second was a sexy coral number with bejeweled netting for the rhumba. We were starting to get noticed for our outfits along with our dancing, and that gave me the confidence to push the envelope a little more. For the third dance, a jive number, I had very specific ideas about what I wanted to wear: a halter top that showed off my neck and collarbones, and an open midriff because my stomach muscles were starting to get so cut from the dancing. I chose hot pink because it's a good color for my skin tone. Louis wanted to do a fringe all over, because it moves really well when you're dancing; I thought the fringe was too long on the skirt and wanted Louis to cut it shorter. The spot where the hem falls on your leg makes all the difference. If it is cut even a little too long, it chops off your legs and makes them look shorter. If the cut is higher, your legs look longer and leaner. Which look do you think I wanted? I was dancing next to Stacy Keibler, who has legs up to her ears. I had to do whatever I could to stand out!

I'll never forget standing backstage, right before the show, telling Louis, "Cut it higher, cut it higher." The fringe was at mid-thigh, and finally I grabbed the scissors and cut it right up to my panty line as Louis was laughing and saying, "No, it's too short!" Clearly, I got my way in the end, and that dress became one of the iconic dresses I wore on the show. They later auctioned it off for charity, and it brought in nearly $20,000. So, that's a good thing!

I've finally learned to trust my gut, and take a risk, and it's paid off in countless ways. I encourage everyone to get out of their comfort zone and take one small risk, which will then lead to taking others in every area of their lives. These risks may not always be successes, but they will always open new doors.

I've also learned, by spending many dollars, that a closet full of clothes doesn't mean you have style. And it certainly doesn't mean you have a *personal* style, which is without a doubt the single most important key to singular style. And like many women, I've bought many a trendy item that didn't go with anything I owned and got tossed out, unworn, after one season. How frustrating is that? Not only is this a waste of your time and money, it does nothing to develop your own personal look, the thing that people think of when they think of you. Items that cultivate your personal look can be tricky to identify at first, but they end up being little things—your personal basics—that define you, such as scarves or funky shoes, or a certain color or cut. For example, I have a friend who never leaves the house without an armful of polished silver bangles. Developing your own signature style will save you tons of time and money in the long run. And remember: less is more when it comes to style and fashion.

A Fun Way to Indulge Expensive Tastes

I get together with three of my girlfriends four times a year to celebrate each of our birthdays. We chip in and buy the birthday girl a great gift, a guilty pleasure that we would never buy for ourselves. Last year, for my forty-fifth birthday, my girlfriends bought me a killer Givenchy clutch from Barneys. It's to die for, and I cherish it because it's from my dearest friends and I never would have bought it for myself. If you and your girlfriends like pricey items, but feel guilty indulging in them, this is a great tradition to adopt. It makes gift giving (and gift getting) so much fun, and there is no buyer's remorse!

I learn a lot by observing what my friends wear—my friends have great style! Twenty-two years ago, I was in an acting class with my friend Lyndie, who is still my best friend to this day. As an acting exercise, we were asked to close our eyes and say what the person next to us was wearing. I was able to describe, in exact detail, the entire outfit

Lyndie had on. I still can today. She was wearing a black off-the-shoulder T-shirt, the coolest hand-painted jeans, Manolo Blahnik flats, and gold hoops. She is one of my style icons and I've always coveted her ability to put things together. When Harry and I were designing the first Belle Gray store, I knew I wanted the interior to look very much like Lyndie's home—all white with dark wood floors and sea grass rugs. Lyndie is a perennial style setter, and her great taste has influenced everyone in our social circle.

I also pick up fashion and style tips from my three birthday girlfriends. Our bodies and personal styles are as different as can be: Lisa T. loves great necklaces, watches, and anything cashmere. Robin is petite and adores Hermès bags; she always wears heels, and her hair and makeup are always perfect (she is also a shopper after my own heart). For her last birthday, we bought Robin a Van Cleef & Arpel clover bracelet. Jana is a stay-at-home mom, with beautiful long blond hair, who loves bandanas, sweatpants, and great unique tops. We bought Jana a Bottega Veneta makeup bag and a Stella McCartney blouse for her last birthday. These are some of the women I have in mind when I buy for my stores.

I love to run around in casual clothes; it's my favorite way to dress and I feel good in my casual wear. And if I'm not confident and comfortable, I just don't function as well. You'll never see me running errands or going to the gym all dolled-up in heels and full makeup; that's not my style and I don't have the time. But you'll also rarely see me in total frump mode because that makes me feel tired and unattractive, and who wants that?

Looking back at how my style has changed over the years, I realized the transformations have been less about my body and more about my age and lifestyle. My body hasn't changed that much over the years. It's my lifestyle that has changed. In my forties, as a wife, mother, and businesswoman, midriff tops and mini-skirts are no-no's!

Funny Fashion Side Note

I was doing a shoot for *Access Hollywood* recently, and the producer asked if I had any photos of me in a bikini in my twenties, thirties, and forties. I did have maybe one bikini photo from my twenties and none from my thirties, but I had *tons* of recent ones from my forties. Since *Dancing with the Stars,* I feel so confident and proud of my body and I love wearing bikinis! Yet I won't wear a midriff top or mini-skirt. Don't get me wrong, I wouldn't parade down Robertson Boulevard in a bikini. But at the beach with my family, I feel it's not only appropriate, it's healthy and good for my daughters to see how comfortable I can be.

It's a different story if I am dressing for the red carpet or a special event—then I like to push the envelope (I call it tapping that Cher factor) and be more daring. I love the whole process of getting ready for awards shows, and I have so much fun doing it. About a month before an event, my stylist, Jen Rade, pulls all kinds of gowns she thinks I might like. She then brings them to my house and I go wild, like a kid in a candy store, trying on dresses all afternoon. Talk about a dream come true—from getting ridiculed for that burgundy sweater dress in Medford, Oregon, to getting paid to wear the most exquisite designs in the world. Lucky me!

Last year, as I was trying on dresses for the Screen Actors Guild awards, Harry happened to be at home while Jen and I were staging our mini-fashion show. When I put on the Jenny Packham leopard-print dress, he said my whole face lit up. Bingo—we had a winner! I had a seamstress take it in a little and when I got it back from her, it was tighter in the bodice and more low-cut, very va-va-voom, complete with a bustier-type bra sewn inside that pushed up my boobs. I figured, why not? That dress got a lot of attention—most of it favorable, thankfully—and it's a good example of the fashion risks I like to take. I don't go out of my way to shock, I just like to have a little fun.

Lisa Rinna Banished!

In the late nineties, Harry and I were dating but not yet married, and his niece was having an engagement party at the Valley Hunt Club in Pasadena, where Harry grew up. Harry was working and couldn't make it, so I was representing the two of us. I'd never been to the club before, and I didn't know where it was or how long it would take to get there, so I ended up arriving early, before any of the other guests had shown up.

The Valley Hunt Club, it turned out, was very "old money," very prim and proper. The women were all in Talbots blazers and pearls. I strode into the main dining room, feeling pretty good about myself in furry, leopard-print, cropped Dolce & Gabbana pants with a black turtleneck. (I thought these pants were the coolest.) As I walked into the dining room, every single person turned around and stared at me; some actually stopped mid-bite, their forks in the air, to gawk. The maitre d' rushed over and told me that women were not allowed in the dining room in pants. Now, this was not the 1950s, it was 1998! He told me I would have to wait for my party upstairs in a separate room. They ushered me upstairs and stuck me in a tiny room that was basically a closet, and closed the door. Not until the rest of the party arrived did they let me out of the room, and then I was admonished again and told that I was not allowed in the dining room.

Did I realize that I wasn't appropriately attired for the venerable Hunt Club? Probably, but I also thought I looked fabulous and stylish, and I do like to push the envelope a little. No harm, no foul, is the way I look at it. And I certainly made an impression! And did I mention that Harry loves this story? He says it's "classic Lisa."

Even when I was pregnant, I always made an effort to look stylish and fashionable. I saw it as a fun challenge. It helped that I felt great and sexy during both of my pregnancies. I loved everything about being pregnant. I didn't have to worry about my body or my weight, and all those pregnancy hormones made my hair and boobs look fabulous. When I was pregnant with my first daughter,

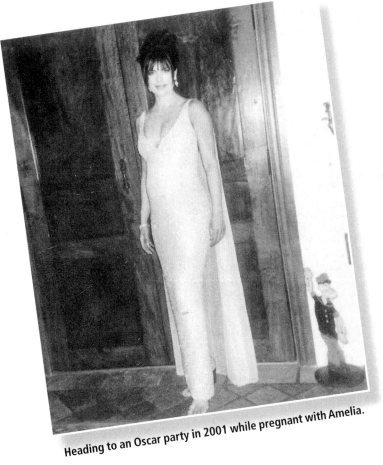

Heading to an Oscar party in 2001 while pregnant with Amelia.

stylish maternity clothes were just starting to be made available. I wore tons of Liz Lange's maternity line, and I never felt I had to sacrifice fashion for comfort or fit.

It's all about making a singular impression. Think "the lady in red." What is your lady in red? If you love wearing jeans, choose the perfect jeans for your body, and find fun tops and accessories to make them fit any occasion.

Though I'm not a big believer in rules when it comes to fashion, I do follow certain guidelines. In general, I wear what makes me feel comfortable and fits my lifestyle, whatever feels appropriate for me at this point (and age) in my life. I stick with the basics—a great pair of jeans, a slim black skirt, a fitted white shirt, a cashmere sweater, a nice watch, a cool pair of sunglasses, and a classic blazer. Fashion is ever-changing, but if you start with the basics, it's easier (and less expensive) to work with the trends. If you're not a fashionista, you're not a fashionista. Don't try to become one. Wear what you feel comfortable in, and what makes you feel good!

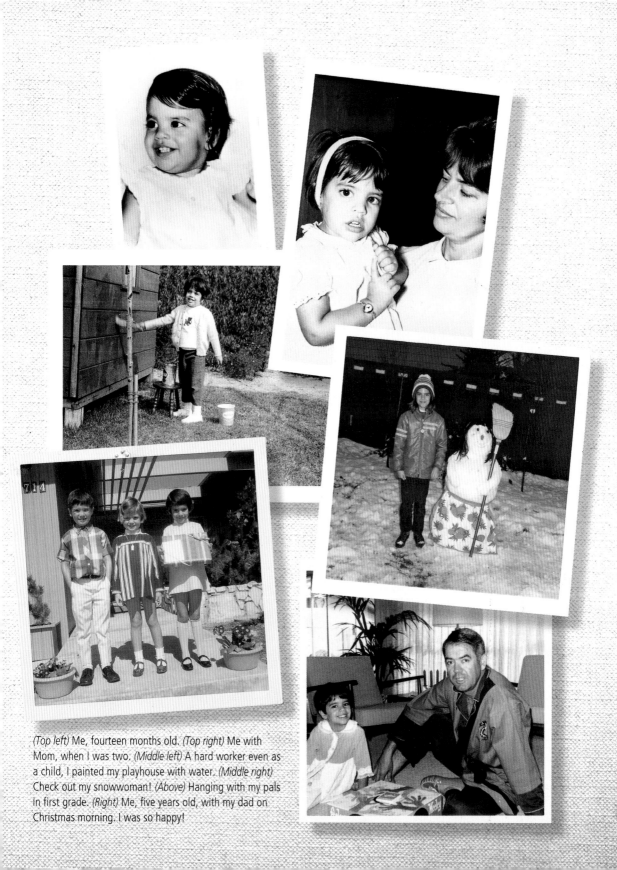

(Top left) Me, fourteen months old. (Top right) Me with Mom, when I was two. (Middle left) A hard worker even as a child, I painted my playhouse with water. (Middle right) Check out my snowwoman! (Above) Hanging with my pals in first grade. (Right) Me, five years old, with my dad on Christmas morning. I was so happy!

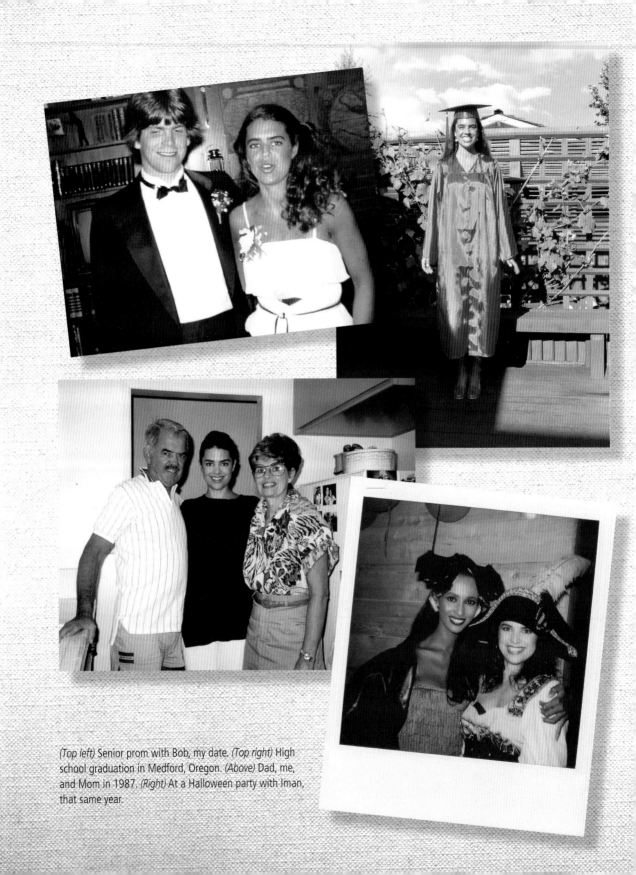

(Top left) Senior prom with Bob, my date. *(Top right)* High
school graduation in Medford, Oregon. *(Above)* Dad, me,
and Mom in 1987. *(Right)* At a Halloween party with Iman,
that same year.

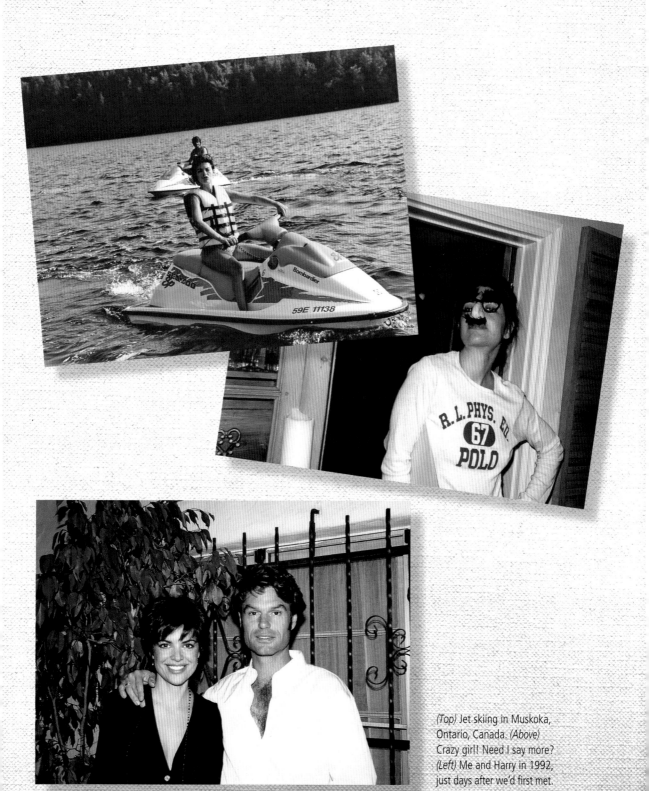

(Top) Jet skiing in Muskoka, Ontario, Canada. (Above) Crazy girl! Need I say more? (Left) Me and Harry in 1992, just days after we'd first met.

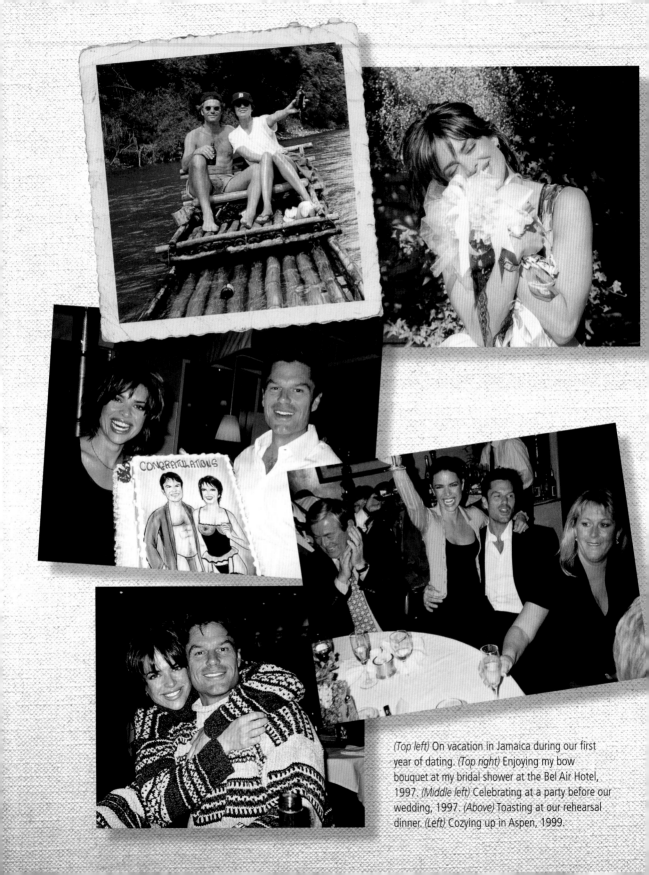

(Top left) On vacation in Jamaica during our first year of dating. *(Top right)* Enjoying my bow bouquet at my bridal shower at the Bel Air Hotel, 1997. *(Middle left)* Celebrating at a party before our wedding, 1997. *(Above)* Toasting at our rehearsal dinner. *(Left)* Cozying up in Aspen, 1999.

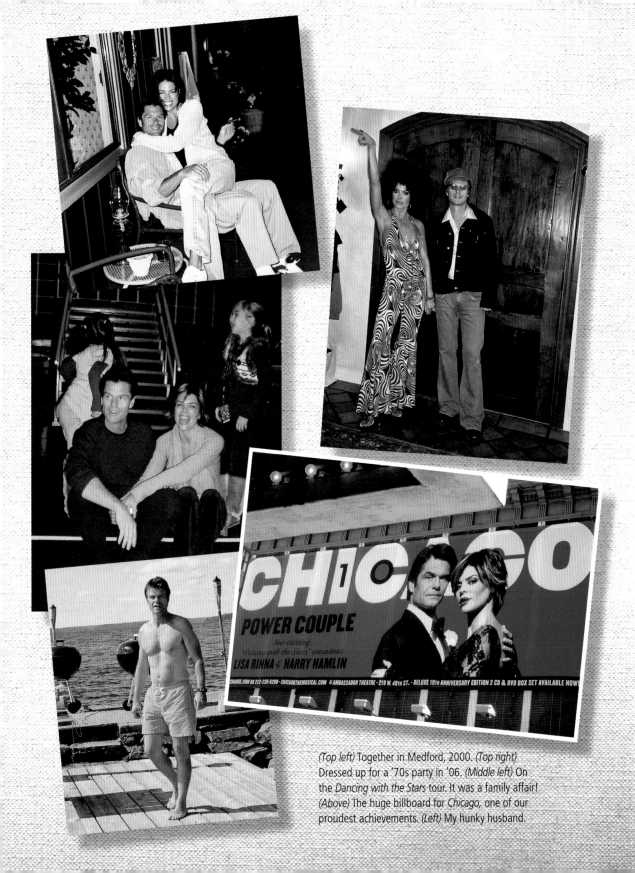

(Top left) Together in Medford, 2000. (Top right) Dressed up for a '70s party in '06. (Middle left) On the Dancing with the Stars tour. It was a family affair! (Above) The huge billboard for Chicago, one of our proudest achievements. (Left) My hunky husband.

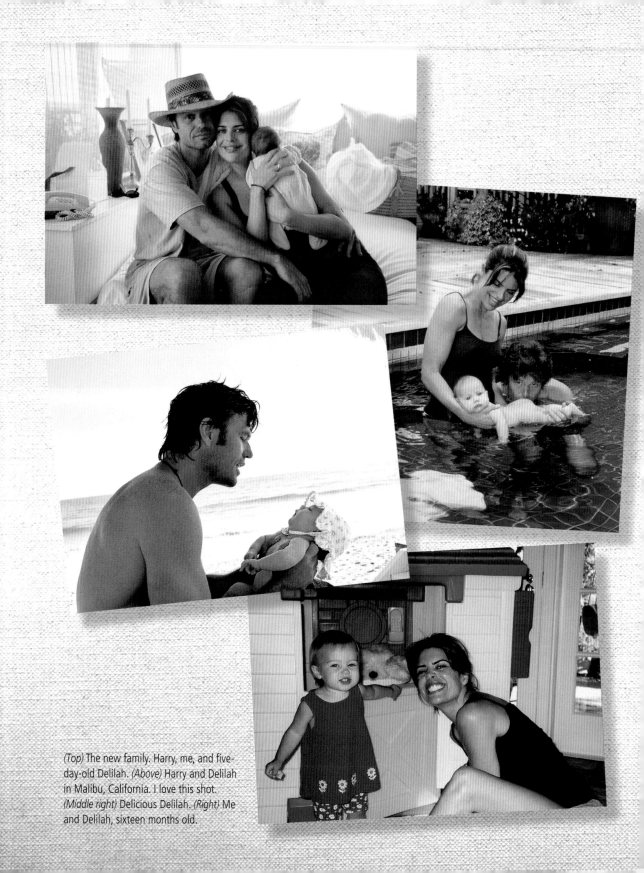

(Top) The new family. Harry, me, and five-day-old Delilah. (Above) Harry and Delilah in Malibu, California. I love this shot. (Middle right) Delicious Delilah. (Right) Me and Delilah, sixteen months old.

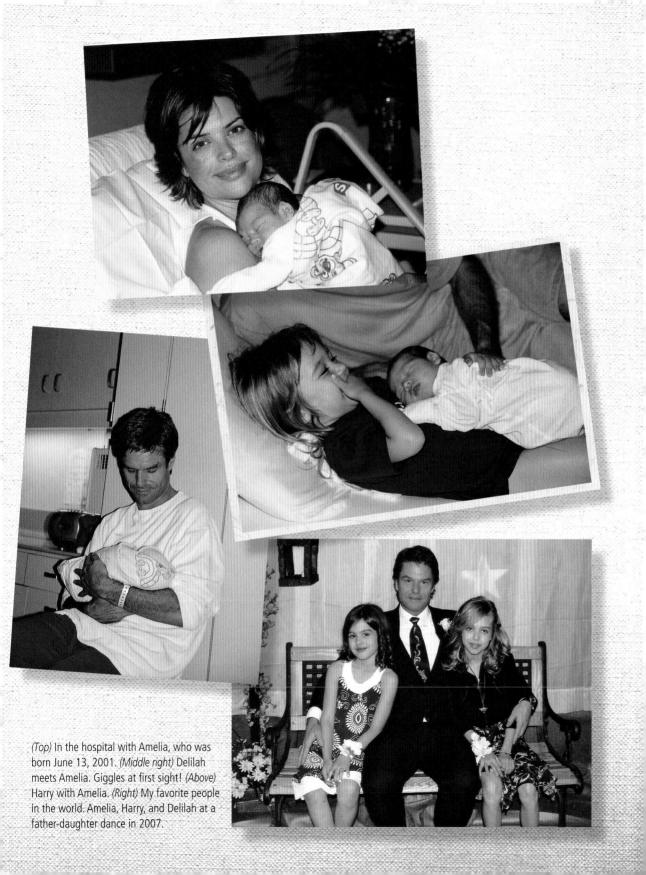

(Top) In the hospital with Amelia, who was born June 13, 2001. *(Middle right)* Delilah meets Amelia. Giggles at first sight! *(Above)* Harry with Amelia. *(Right)* My favorite people in the world. Amelia, Harry, and Delilah at a father-daughter dance in 2007.

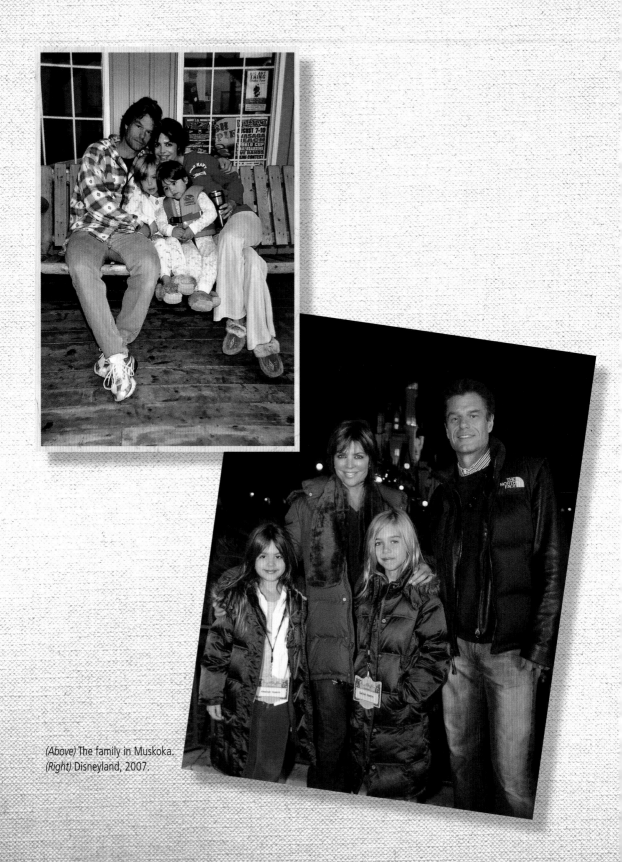

(*Above*) The family in Muskoka.
(*Right*) Disneyland, 2007.

My Top Ten Favorite Things in My Closet

These are things I could never part with. Most of them I have had for years. Some have sentimental value and all run the gamut in price:

- Yves Saint Laurent leopard bag

- Ray-Ban black aviator shades that I wear everywhere

- Converse silver sneakers that dress up even the most casual outfit

- Gucci knee-length black leather jacket

- An Azzedine Alaia black lace bustier gown that Harry bought for me fifteen years ago and that I still wear

- JET wide-legged jeans that I wear going out or running around doing errands—I had them hemmed to a very versatile length.

- Levi's 501 boy-cut jeans that are my hanging out/running errand jeans. I think of them as my "kid-friendly jeans," since I can bend over in them and not worry about anything showing!

- Havianas pewter flip-flops, which are perfect for running around in.

- C&C black T-shirts (C&C was one of the first clothing lines I carried at Belle Gray, and it is still one of my top sellers). These are a must-have staple for me.

- A taupe silk scarf my best friend Lyndie brought me from India. I wear it with everything, and it adds a boho-cool vibe to any outfit.

My Most Memorable Fashion Moments

Since I've said I can clock my life through fashion, I've put together a timeline of my favorite events:

- **1992**—white Gucci gown by Tom Ford (Carousel Ball). This is the first expensive gown I bought myself. It cost $1,300. I was sick to my stomach when I signed the receipt!

- **1994**—black Versace cutout gown (Carousel Ball). Another expensive dress I bought myself. This one was $2,000, and I was just as sick about the purchase, but I had to buy it—no designer would loan me a dress.

- **1996**—yellow dress—the designer escapes me—slit up the side (American Music Awards). This was very risqué for me.

- **1997**—Azzedine Alaia black lace dress that Harry bought me. This is my favorite dress ever. It's so sexy and chic. I wore it to the Soap Opera Digest Awards, and Robert Kelker-Kelley and I won for "Best Couple."

- **2000**—red, sparkly Giorgio Armani dress (Daytime Emmys). This was a gorgeous halter-neck dress. So flashy and fun.

- **2001**—white Reem Acra (Daytime Emmys). I was a presenter that year, and I had been nominated for my hosting role on *Soaptalk*.

- **2002**—nude Vera Wang (Daytime Emmys). That year I was nominated for "Best Host" and for "Best Talk Show" for *Soaptalk*.

- **2005**—Narciso Rodriguez blue gown (Daytime Emmys). I was once again nominated for "Best Talk Show Host" and "Best Talk Show" for *Soaptalk*.
- **2006**—pink-fringed jive dress (*Dancing with the Stars* Season Two). So fun!
- **2006**—Pamela Dennis leopard-print dress (Hollyrod, Holly Robinson Peete's annual event to raise money to fight Parkinson's disease). Who doesn't love leopard print?
- **2007**—Reem Acra red dress (Daytime Emmys). I was nominated for "Best Host" for *Soaptalk*.
- **2007**—Elsie Katz dress (Golden Globe Awards). Gorgeous!
- **2008** (January)—leopard-print Jenny Packham dress (SAG Awards). I fell in love with this dress, which I wore while doing red-carpet commentary for TV Guide Network.
- **2008**—silver Hervé Léger (Grammy Awards). I wore this sexy number while doing commentary on the red carpet for TV Guide Network.
- **2008**—navy Reem Acra strapless dress (Academy Awards). I felt so glamorous while doing red-carpet commentary for TV Guide Network in this gown.
- **2008**—gorgeous one-shoulder Reem Acra gown (Emmys). Loved it!
- **2009**—I'll never forget the beaded black-and-white Reem Acra halter I wore to the Golden Globes.
- **2009**—black one-shoulder Zuhair Murad (Grammys).
- **2009**—red Pamela Rolland (SAG Awards). Such a good dress!

As I always say, fashion is all about taking risks and expressing yourself. I love classic black, white, and neutrals, but I also love bright colors and patterns, and of course, I adore animal prints. I say that my fashion model is Jackie O meets Kate Moss with a little Cher or Tina Turner thrown in—classic, simple style with a little bit of wildness.

I also love the bohemian look—think Kate Hudson (and her mom, Goldie), Sienna Miller, and Kate Moss. When I want to emulate their style, I look for funky, colorful clothes and bold jewelry, anything vintage that gives that laid-back but still chic vibe. A great look is a pair of boyfriend jeans and a peasant top with dangly earrings and thong sandals. I also like peasant-style tunic dresses with bare legs and killer sandals, or tights and boots.

Take It from Me: Three Key Fashion Tips I've Learned Over the Years

1. FINDING THE BEST JEANS FOR YOUR BODY TYPE

Today, jeans come in every price range and a cut to fit any body. Remember when it was either classic Levi's or high-waisted "mom" jeans? On the positive side, those days are over, but the number of choices out there can be overwhelming. You *have* to try them on to see what flatters you. I know it can be a trying experience, but it's the only way to find the perfect pair. Take a friend whose opinion you trust, go to a store with a good selection, and don't leave until you've found them. My favorites are Levi's 501 boy-cut jeans and any boot-leg style because they make my legs look longer and they seem to fit my body type well.

2. GETTING YOUR SEXY ON

Deep down, we all know what's sexy and what's not. But sometimes everyday life gets in the way, and suddenly your daily uniform is an old T-shirt and saggy sweat-pants. When that happens, it's time to get your sexy back on! Sexy is about feeling comfortable in your own skin. I don't consciously try to dress sexy. I wear what I like and what looks good on me; if it happens to show a little skin, that's okay, and if I look sexy, all the better!

Most of the time, less is more, simpler is sexier. Harry likes me best in a T-shirt and jeans with little or no makeup. The look is fun and relaxed, and it shows I'm there with him and the kids—I'm present and not worrying about how I look, or who is going to see me. Now the T-shirt isn't a midriff top or a baggy hand-me-down from Harry, and the jeans aren't skin-tight and ripped to shreds and patched-up, but it is a look that makes me feel good and playful, and that translates to sexiness.

Figure out what makes you feel attractive and open to having fun. It can be a sundress, a pair of cute shorts with a button-down, whatever—put it on whenever you feel like you spend too much time in your usual uniform.

3. DEVELOPING SIGNATURE TOUCHES

I love hoop earrings in gold or silver, or with diamonds, both fancy and casual. I wear them so often that my friends consider them my signature style of jewelry.

In addition to my hoop earrings, sunglasses are another signature accessory. Tom Ford, Gucci, and Ray-Ban aviator-style glasses are my favorite. They hide a multitude of sins—when I have under-eye bags, puffiness, or I'm running around with no makeup on.

I find that scarves are incredibly versatile, and a great way to cozy up any outfit. They can be wrapped around your hair or tied around your neck. If, like Nora Ephron, your neck makes you feel bad, use scarves to cover your neck or décolletage. (I tend to break out on my chest, so a scarf can be a lifesaver.) If you have on a more casual outfit, wind a big scarf around your neck a few times, or use a scarf as a headband, Jackie O. style. Finish it off with big sunglasses, and all of a sudden you're transformed into a woman with style. I think every woman should invest in one quality cashmere shawl—they last forever and never go out of style.

My Must-Have Accessories

- A great cashmere shawl
- A good black or camel-colored coat, preferably cashmere
- A fabulous pair of designer sunglasses
- A gorgeous pair of Christian Louboutin high heels
- A pair of high-heeled leather boots
- A pair of cowboy boots to wear with jeans or dresses
- A great bag—it doesn't have to be expensive. I recently bought an inexpensive chocolate-brown leather bag with pockets on the side, and I get tons of compliments on it.

Belle Gray

While the seeds for opening my own boutique were planted as far back as 2000, it wasn't until December of 2001 that they began to take root. Harry was appearing at an event in Rancho Santa Fe, near San Diego, and I had gone along with him. While he was busy working, I had time on my hands and decided to do what I do best—shop. I wandered into a store called Gracie Boutique. The minute I walked through the door, I fell in love. It had the cutest mix of clothes, all of my favorite designer labels, and it was all of 600 square feet (which is tiny!). I immediately thought, *This is the kind of store I want to open.*

Though I already had the idea for the store, so far it was just a concept I was toying with in the back of my mind. I began chatting with the owner, Gracie Mahvi, and then I started asking her questions—how did she choose the clothes for her store? How did she go about ordering them?—pretty basic questions, since I had absolutely no retail experience beyond my after-school job at the Lerner's department store in Medford, but Gracie was so incredibly generous with her time and knowledge, and answered everything. She also told me the first thing I needed to do was to go into my closet at home and write down the names of the lines I liked.

Upon returning home to LA, I sat on the floor of my closet, yellow legal pad in hand, and made a list of the label names I preferred and what I like about them: Theory button-down shirts and trousers, Diane von Furstenberg dresses; James Perse California-style basics, Vince sweaters, C&C T-shirts, and so on until I had a complete list that would fill a store. Gracie knew what she was talking about—the names I wrote on my pad that day are consistently my top sellers even now. Gracie also introduced me to the market centers—the California Mart and the New Mart in particular—in downtown Los Angeles, where all the shop owners go four times a year to see what's hot and get an inside track on the new fashions.

Unfortunately, not every shop owner was as gracious as Gracie. If I thought show biz was tough, I hadn't seen anything yet. The boutique owners were very territorial, and did not like newcomers encroaching on their turf. When I tried to stock my beloved James Perse clothes, I discovered that *I wasn't allowed to* because a boutique down the street had an exclusive on his line in that area. Do you believe how naïve I was? I really had no idea. I was definitely made to feel unwelcome; but by this point, I was in it for the long haul, and I stuck to my guns and did what I had to do to set up my dream store. In the process, I endured many sleepless nights. We were basically flying blind those first few years. With no formal fashion training or retail experience, all I had to go on was my own taste and style. It took a while for us to hit our stride, to win the vendors over, and to build a loyal customer base. But it was worth it in the end.

These days, Belle Gray is a one-stop shopping experience. We sell candles, lingerie, clothing, shoes, and jewelry. We dress women from age ten to eighty, and we can dress anyone for any event—we have customers coming in who need something for a night on the town, a reunion, a wedding, a weekend getaway, a movie premiere, or their child's school play; and they rarely leave empty-handed. Our website, www.bellegray.com, designed by Harry, has also been successful, thank goodness, and we get orders from all over the country. If I sound like a proud mother, I am. The name Belle Gray comes from our daughters' middle names—Delilah Belle and Amelia Gray—and these stores are our babies too. We have shops in Sherman Oaks and Calabasas in California. Along with our amazing daughters, Belle Gray is one of Harry's and

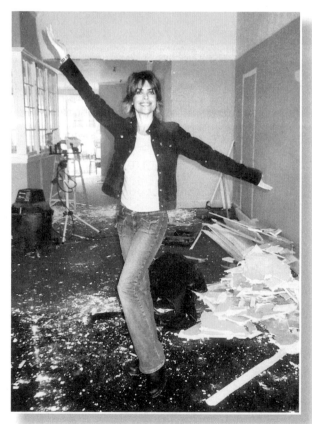

The very beginning of Belle Gray . . .

my proudest accomplishments. It's a result of one of my passions; it's led me to meet tons of great new people, I've learned volumes about the business, and it's something I created with Harry.

You might not love to play dress-up as much as I do. Hey, you might not even like to shop! I understand that not everyone shares my passion for fashion, but I encourage everyone to be open to the power of a great outfit that can help you feel confident and attractive and transform you a tiny bit every time you put it on. A little Rinnavation can be as simple as a little black dress.

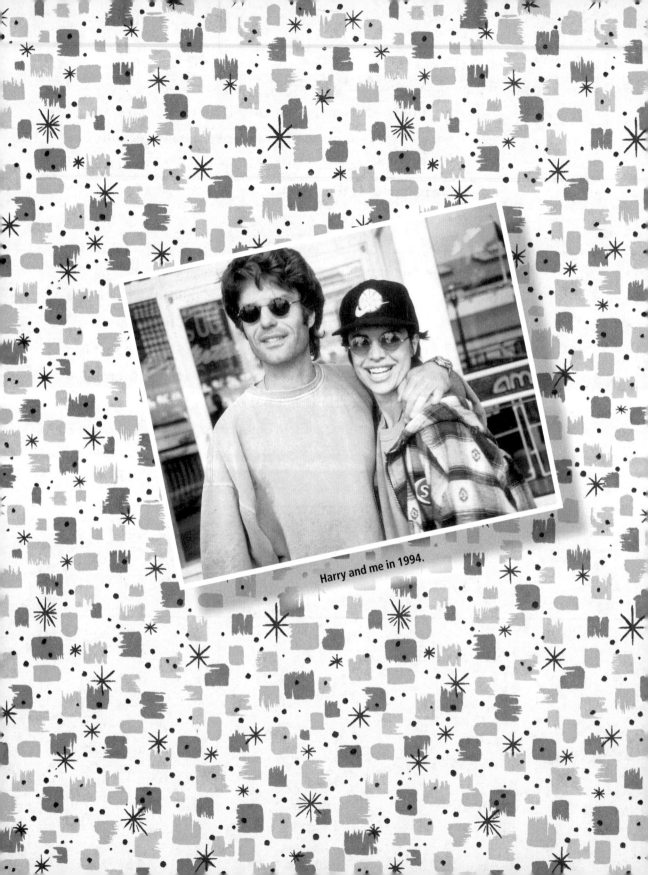

Harry and me in 1994.

HAPPY WIFE, HAPPY LIFE: MARRIAGE AND SEX

A great marriage is not when the "perfect couple" comes together. It is when an imperfect couple learns to enjoy their differences.

—DAVE MEURER, *DAZE OF OUR WIVES*

Marriage

There's a story that Harry and I love to tell that perfectly captures our relationship. A few years ago, after being together for over a decade, we were on vacation in a small lakeside town, and we stumbled upon an old-fashioned candy store that had all kinds of candies we remembered from childhood. Harry told me Jujubes were his favorite candy and that he loved the purple ones. "The purple ones are my favorite too!" I yelled. And we proceeded to discuss our intense love of Jujubes. It was the first thing we had ever had in common.

It's true, you couldn't find two people more opposite than Harry and I. Fortunately, in our case, opposites do attract, and we complement each other's strengths and weaknesses. But practically everything about us is as different as night and day. Harry was raised in affluent Pasadena, California, attended private schools, and went to college at Berkeley and Yale. Everything always came easy to him. After the success of his film *Clash of the Titans*, he was in such demand that he found himself saying no to most offers, including a major contract from Warner Brothers (of course I would have died for a chance like that!). He still turns things down today. I, on the other hand, grew up middle-class, in Medford. I had to fight for every single thing I've gotten in my life, and still do. My motto has always been, *The answer is yes; now what's the question?* Luckily, we totally click.

I'm convinced I met Harry exactly when I was supposed to. Any earlier, and I wouldn't have been ready for him, and I certainly wouldn't have appreciated him. I first had to go through a series of relationships to find out what I wanted and what I didn't want. I was twenty-nine years old when I met Harry in 1992, and pretty much an emotional mess. I had never allowed myself to be treated nicely by a man. I didn't respect or love myself enough to feel I deserved a great relationship.

Turning Your Differences into Strengths

Every six months or so, I have a strategy meeting with my agents. We get together and go over a list of projects that might be worth pursuing. During one meeting in early 2007, we saw that the TV Guide Network was looking for a "couple" to host the red carpet. Immediately, my agent thought Harry and I would be perfect! My agents pitched it to the TV Guide Network executives, who liked the idea, so we set up a meeting. Harry, however, had no interest in the project. At the meeting with the programming executives, Harry was "selling" me big-time. Though he had no desire to do the show, and didn't even want to be in the meeting, he thought I was perfect for the job, and he knew that if he got into the room with them he could sell them on the idea of just me and not him (at the same time, I was trying to sell *him* big-time, and he was practically kicking me under the table!). A few weeks later, the executives called my agent and very gingerly said, "We love Lisa and would love to hire her, but we don't think Harry is the right fit." Needless to say, Harry jumped up and down for joy (one thing I'd never seen him do before, by the way!), and I did too.

People are always surprised when I tell them I had only five lovers before Harry. All but two were long-term relationships that endured long after they should have. My first boyfriend, to whom I lost my virginity when I was sixteen, was named Todd. We were together for a year or so until I saw him out with another girl.

After Todd came Bob, and my longest relationship—eight and a half years—until Harry. We were inseparable: where one went the other one followed. He followed me to Emerson College in Boston, and then I followed Bob to the University of Oregon. When Bob got a job in San Francisco, I followed him there, where I began teaching at the Richard Simmons studio. We were like an old married couple, or a brother and sister. I stayed because it was comfortable, and I was afraid to go out on my own. The entire three and a half years we lived in San Francisco, I was miserable. Bob worked long hours, and I didn't have any friends. Eventually I met some women through the exercise studio, and we would have weekly *Dynasty*-watching parties. Little did I know that ten years later I would be on an Aaron Spelling show, *Melrose Place*! I wasn't yet acting, and didn't feel good about myself because I didn't feel I was accomplishing anything. After I convinced Bob that we should move to Los Angeles, I finally started to find my groove. I was getting work in commercials, taking acting classes, and meeting lots of people. The relationship ended when I began an affair with Peter, an actor who was working on a soap opera.

I was twenty-five years old when I became involved with Peter, and my relationship with him lasted three and a half years. It was the worst relationship and time of my life. I cried every single day, because Peter couldn't give me what I needed, and I beat myself up about it. He was a commitment-phobe; to this day he is a confirmed bachelor. He was emotionally unavailable and cheap. In our time together, he rarely bought me dinner—we would split the check. Big warning bells should have gone off the very first time I went to his apartment. Peter was a former model, incredibly gorgeous, in great physical shape, and meticulous about his appearance. His home was an entirely different matter. He was a total pack rat, and there were clothes strewn over every surface, in every corner. It always looked like someone had just ransacked the place. And I just totally accepted it! I must have attracted this relationship because of how I felt about myself at the time. I was so desperate to be loved. Then there was the little matter of not being able to sleep in his bed. I never did, not once, in three and a half years. It was my choice; I couldn't sleep in the same bed with him. I would get insomnia and not be able to fall asleep (hello, warning bells). If I stayed overnight, I would sleep on the couch. Mind you, I am not trying to play the victim and make him the villain. I created this situation by choosing him and staying with him. No one was forcing me; it was my choice. Now when I look back on it, I cannot believe that I was that person, but in the end Peter turned out to be one of my greatest teachers.

The relationship with Peter ended when I had an affair with an actor six years my junior. (I call him my "boy-toy fling"). Having an affair was my way of ending a relationship. After sharing an apartment with my friend Joel for three years, I finally decided I had to be on my own, to live alone. It was one of those gut instincts that paid off. Eight months later, I met Harry. He was as gun-shy as I was. He was coming off a bad marriage and a dysfunctional relationship prior to that, and had zero interest in getting married again. I knew I needed to give him space. I sensed that he was a good guy, and worth the wait. We dated for five years before we got married, but we've been best friends and soul mates since we first met sixteen years ago. We just had to realize it at our own pace.

Despite our differences, we have the important stuff in common. We share the same values, and the same commitment to marriage and family. Our past relationships taught us a lot, and mutually acknowledging that and being open about it created an immediate bond and a mutual respect. We know from hard-won experience how hard, and rare, it is to have a happy, healthy relationship, so we never take ours for granted. And we're both in it for the long haul. Our commitment to each other and our marriage is rooted in a philosophy I've developed over the years: I believe we all have a choice about how we perceive things, and the way we react to them. I've learned to try not to focus on the bad things or the little stuff, or what could go wrong. Instead, I try to look at the good things, and the big picture. If I think the worst, that's what will happen. But if I think

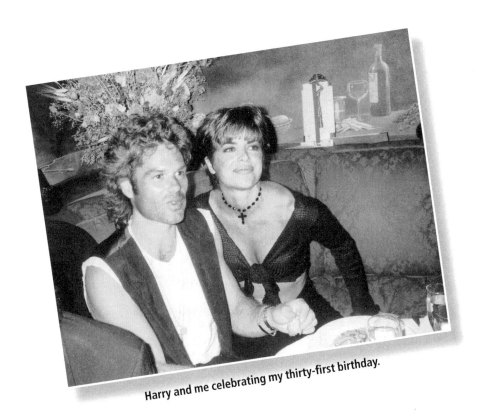

Harry and me celebrating my thirty-first birthday.

everything's going to turn out great, it will. Granted, it's not always that black and white. In every relationship, there are compromises and sacrifices each person must be willing to make—things that can make or break a relationship. Trust me, Harry and I have both done our share of compromising, especially early on in our relationship when we were both so wounded and guarded. But eventually, we were able to overcome our fears and baggage; and now our relationship stands on that strong foundation.

In addition to staying positive and being willing to give a little bit now and then, Harry and I work because we support each other in everything we do. So, of course, when I was doing *Dancing with the Stars*, Harry was my biggest fan and cheerleader. He would rub my feet and comfort me when I came home exhausted after a day of practice. He was in the audience for every one of my performances, and the cameras caught the emotion on his face as I performed. You could feel that he was totally there with me, body, mind, and spirit, and I was totally there for him when he did *Dancing with the Stars* the following season. In fact, Harry decided to do *Dancing with the Stars* (something very far outside his usual comfort zone) because he wanted to experience what I had. He wanted us to be connected through that life-changing experience. I am in awe of him for doing it.

The Keys to a Successful Relationship, Learned Through Experience

I've found that the best ways to strengthen and sustain your relationship are to respect each other at all times, treat your partner the way that you want to be treated, and take time out for your relationship by planning moments where you and your partner can be alone with each other (yes, this does require *planning*). It's really that simple.

We've also learned to capitalize on our differences by turning them into strengths. In fact, as partners in business, our differences are huge assets. I am the emotional, impetuous one. Harry is intellectual, thoughtful, and considered in his approach. When I met him, I thought he was the most intimidating person I had ever met. Unlike me, it takes him a while to warm up to people. It's not that he's standoffish or cold. He is just very deliberate, very intense, and ironically, completely oblivious to how intimidating he can be.

When we were opening the first Belle Gray store, he drew up the plans for the store, handled all the financial details, and automatically assumed all the chief operating duties. I chose the clothing lines and learned the ropes of the fashion retail world. Soon after we opened the store, we learned that Oprah was going to feature Belle Gray on her annual show dedicated to showcasing celebrities' favorite places to go. We were only three months old and we didn't even have a website. Therefore, we were not going to be able to capitalize on the great publicity. Harry, coolly and calmly, went to the bookstore and bought a copy of *Websites for Dummies*. A few weeks later, we had our website, which was a good thing, since right after the show aired, we got 770,000 hits per minute (!) and thousands of dollars in orders. I can pick out all of the clothes in the world, but if Harry's not watching the store, the business will go down the tubes (which, by the way, it almost has at least three times since we opened our first Belle Gray).

Our differences also become strengths in terms of major decision making. I tend to go by my gut, and usually don't stop to weigh the pros and cons. If it feels right, I go for it. For example, when I was pregnant with our daughter Delilah, I had the idea to pose for *Playboy* (crazy, I know). Harry thought it was a bad idea. I gave him all the reasons I thought it was a great idea, and eventually he came around. I love that he doesn't just dig in his heels and refuse to budge. He really listens and considers all sides of an argument before he makes up his mind. We are each other's sounding board; we make every decision together. If something works, we both reap the benefits. If it doesn't, we take the hit together.

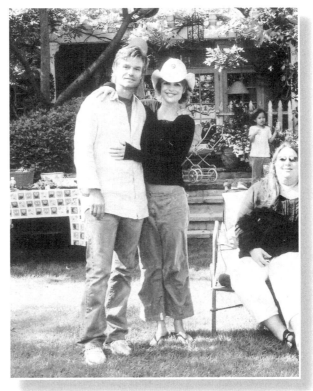

Harry and me hosting a party in our backyard.

Now, sixteen years into our relationship, I see us less as opposites, and more like each other's alter ego. I help him lighten up a little, and he makes me more grounded and less emotional. Plain and simple, we bring out the best in each other. At the end of the day, isn't that what a partnership is all about? I believe our marriage works because Harry and I respect each other and we never forget that. It's the key to staying together, we think. (Well, there's also the great sex, but I'll get to that later.)

Astrologically Matched

A friend e-mailed me these horoscopes. They couldn't be more true!

- **Cancer**—the Protector (Lisa): Moody, emotional. May be shy. Very loving and caring. Pretty/handsome. Excellent partner for life. Protective. Inventive and imaginative. Cautious. Touchy-feely kind of person. Needs love from others. Easily hurt, but sympathetic.
- **Scorpio**—the Intense One (Harry): Very energetic. Intelligent. Can be jealous and/or possessive. Hardworking. Great kisser. Can become obsessive or secretive. Holds grudges. Attractive. Determined. Loves being in long-term relationships. Talkative. Romantic. Can be self-centered at times. Passionate and emotional.

Let's Talk About Sex

Harry and I had been dating about a year when my best friend told me she had recently attended a "sex education party" hosted by an incredible woman. She said that it had been highly enlightening (and not nearly as awkward as one might think). Game as always to try something new, I hosted a party at my house for a bunch of my girlfriends. The "sexpert," Lou Paget, was just as amazing as my friend had said. Lou teaches women all the tricks of the trade, and demystifies the art and science of pleasing your man. Her expertise comes from a fail-proof source: years before, she had asked her gay friend to teach her everything he knew about technique—right down to step-by-step instructions. Obviously, she was a stellar pupil, and eventually, she began teaching what she'd learned to groups of women in people's homes—sort of Tupperware parties for sex ed.

So there we were, a group of eight women, assembled in my living room giggling nervously because we had no idea what to expect. Lou came in, and she couldn't have been less like a typical Tupperware saleslady. A Beverly Hills blonde, she is thin and elegant with impeccable hair and clothes, but also incredibly engaging and professional. She put us immediately at ease (well, she and a few glasses of wine). The first thing she did was pull out a big bag of rubber penises, in every shape, size, and color. She lined them up in the dishwasher and sterilized them, and we each had to pick one. Then she had us stick them to a plate for easy maneuvering. She proceeded to explain to us, in great detail and with no embarrassment, how to give the best hand and blow jobs (best things I ever learned! I truly believe that knowing how to give a great hand job and an amazing blow job are two very important things every woman should know). It was all very clinical. She would critique each of us as we were practicing, just as a yoga instructor would during class. I don't think I will ever forget the image of my best friend with a penis in her mouth, receiving tips from Lou and making adjustments! The party is definitely the closest I will ever get to group sex, and my friends and I giggled and howled. It was priceless!

Afterwards, Harry was very eager to see what I had learned. (Men love these parties because you're learning to make them happy. Duh!) Like the S Factor strip class I would discover later, Lou's class completely changed my attitude toward sex and my relationship with Harry. I have always been wildly attracted to him, but I had my hang-ups. Now I had more confidence, and skills, to really let loose. Whenever someone says, "You do that?!" I reply, "He's my husband." It's not like I am picking up strange men in bars and honing my techniques on them. This is the father of my children, my best friend, my soul mate for life, and the best lover I've ever had. If I can't go there with him, then we have a big problem.

One thing that struck me after taking that class is how few couples have great, or even good, sex lives. We as women are socialized to think sex is somehow shameful or unladylike. Even in this day and age! Add to that the fact that men and women are wired completely differently when it comes to sex, and it's no wonder most people are doing without, or seeking it elsewhere. I think it's an incredible shame. There is absolutely no better way to connect with your partner on every level.

The Seal and the Ring

This is a great technique I learned from Lou. Basically, it is the first and most important step to giving great oral sex.

Form the Seal by closing your thumb and index finger around your mouth like you're making the "okay" sign. Then with your thumb and forefinger, tighten and release the pressure. This, known as the Ring, controls how deeply the penis enters your mouth. By using the Seal and the Ring, you can create a deep-throat sensation without taking the entire penis into your mouth (this move also prevents gagging).

Continue to let your hands help you. Use your Seal and Ring hand to twist the shaft. And don't forget "the stepchildren" (Lou's term for the testicles, as they tend to be ignored). With your free hand, fondle or stroke his testicles *very lightly*.

And remember, technique is important, as you don't want to hurt anything (cover those teeth!), but enthusiasm and willingness are just as important. Your partner's response will give you all the encouragement you need.

That class with Lou was the beginning of my sexual evolution. I wasn't as afraid of letting loose anymore. My approach to sex is now like my approach to life—you grow and develop by learning from experience, facing your fears, and finding out what you like and don't like. And, as with exercise and fashion, I can track the stages of my life through the steps of my sexual evolution.

Like most women, through the years, I've occasionally needed little tune-ups to get the juices flowing again. After I had my daughter Delilah, I was feeling completely un-sexual, dried-up, and depressed. Lou's famous "basket" technique (which I'll share later in this chapter) was a far and distant memory. The sexual spark in me had gone out. Luckily, I had stumbled across an article in the *Los Angeles Times* about Sheila Kelley and her S Factor classes. I was intrigued and, knowing I had nothing to lose, I signed up for a session. I knew if I didn't get my mojo back I would never feel like a sexual being again, and I was going to lose my husband. That was the last thing I wanted. Why do you think some men go to hookers or have affairs? So I said to myself, *Why don't you be the hooker*? The classes brought my sexuality back, and they also turned out to be a fantastic motivator. When you look and feel great, you feel more sexy and sensual. And the increased stamina and strength you get from the classes don't hurt either!

I believe you have to play (notice I didn't say *work*) to keep your sex life alive. I wear sexy lingerie and dress up in costumes—maid, nurse, you name it. I dance and strip for Harry. My philosophy is I can't cook, I'm no good at cleaning my house, but I can service my husband in the bedroom. For most men, sex is more important than putting food on the table anyway. But the main reason my husband is so happy is because *I am willing* to be sexy and sexual. That, in a nutshell, is the secret, ladies. Letting your man know you are attracted to him, and willing and eager to go there—anywhere—with him is an incredible turn-on. Harry couldn't care less that I burn spaghetti and can't work the vacuum. I joke that all any woman needs to do to please her man is walk into the room and bend over. I think we've all forgotten what it's like to be eighteen years old and crazy for someone. Everyday life intrudes, and passion and intimacy end up way down on the list of priorities. You need to make it interesting, make it as fun and as wild as you want. A healthy sex life is all about keeping things fresh and exciting, and pleasing your partner.

If you're not quite up to doing the "walk in/bend over" move yet, try creating a romantic evening for your partner. Trust me, on the surface, you may be doing it for him, but you will get so much in return. Don't over-think things, but make a date, go away somewhere, and let loose. Get out of your house and away from the kids and the pets and the everyday distractions of life and be with your partner. Our house is extremely chaotic—Harry and I are busy, and the kids are always running around—and managing to have sex can seem nearly impossible. So Harry and I schedule nights away at a hotel every two to three months—whenever we seem to feel it's time to reconnect and be intimate. It really keeps us together and connected.

If you can't manage to plan an entire getaway or even a romantic evening, try something spontaneous: buy a sexy negligee or rent a sexy movie. Harry and I love to watch sexy videos. I admit it, I like to watch erotic movies with my husband. It may seem intimidating at first, but it's fun, and it works—it gets us going after sixteen years together. Do what feels comfortable to you!

Trust me, ladies. I know that sometimes it takes nothing short of a boob job to get your mojo back.

In fact, that's exactly what it took for me to feel sexual again six years ago.

Harry and I had decided to spend a night at the St. Regis Hotel in Dana Point, California, as a little romantic getaway. However, despite the perfect setting and my intention to do everything possible to set the right mood, I was not able to be sexual with Harry. Even after having taken striptease classes, I couldn't shake the feeling of being asexual! I was feeling bad about myself and couldn't figure out why, so instead of spending the evening doing anything remotely romantic, I took my insecurities and frustrations out on Harry and picked a fight. In the midst of my tirade, I blurted out, "I just don't feel sexy with my ski-slope, sucked-out boobs!" Harry just looked at me incredulously.

That was it! One huge reason I didn't feel sexual after the birth of my second daughter was because my boobs were shot. I had always had small, perky boobs that I'd felt good about, but after having two kids, no amount of exercise in the world was going to bring them back. I wanted to feel like a woman again—I wanted to have my nice boobs back, and I knew how to get them.

Harry said, "No way. Don't do it. I love you just the way you are." But I knew it was something I needed to do to feel like a sexual person again. I *had* to do it. I know that sounds very superficial, but sometimes making a change to your outside helps you feel better on the inside, and I needed help.

So I found the best boob guy in town and he gave me some good ones. And, for the record, I did get Harry to come around to the idea before I went through with it, and I know he would agree that my boob job was a good decision—it made me feel like a woman again and resuscitated our sex life!

Being open to trying new things and discussing sex has completely rejuvenated my sex life, and I urge you to open up too. Hey, I've even discussed my sex life on *The Howard Stern Show*. Howard and I were kidding around for a while at the beginning of the interview. He gave me some advice on my red-carpet hosting, and then, this being Howard, the conversation turned to sex. He asked me about my sex life with Harry, and without thinking, I just told the truth. I wasn't trying to be coy or cute. I laid it out there. And Howard was shocked!

I told him about Lou Paget's sex party and some of the techniques I had learned. Not one person in that room knew what the "basket" was, but they begged me to tell them! He asked me if Harry and I watched porn together, and if we ever went to strip clubs. I said, "Yes, of course!" I told him about dressing up and stripping for Harry— the whole nine yards. And you know what? It felt great to talk about my great sex life with my husband. In my twenties and thirties, I never would have had the nerve to be so honest. But now I am proud of my sexuality and my relationship with my husband, and I don't feel embarrassed. In fact, on air with Howard, I felt I was lifting some of the taboos about sex, and encouraging people to let go of their fear, to get out of their comfort zones, and to try something new. That show and the response to it were incredibly freeing. Thanks, Howard!

The Amazing Basket Technique

- **Step 1:** Apply lubricant to both hands.
- **Step 2:** Clasp your hands together, interlacing your fingers.
- **Step 3:** Relax your thumbs, forming a hole between your thumbs and your forefingers.
- **Step 4:** Lower your clasped hands onto his penis. The fit should be snug. (In essence, you are creating an "impostor" vagina.)
- **Step 5:** Move your clasped hands up and down the shaft, maintaining a firm yet gentle hold.
- **Step 6:** Twist your clasped hands slowly as they go up and down the shaft, much like the movement inside a washing machine. Use one long twist per shaft length, not a quick swishing back and forth.

Don't get me wrong. I know from experience that getting back in the saddle can be tough. Rarely do both partners want to have sex at the same time. Here's a tip: try to think about it as though you were going to the gym, or attending a social event. Often, you dread going, but once you get there you're glad you did, and you feel great afterwards. For most of us, psyching ourselves up for sex is all about shutting off those voices in our heads, hiding our to-do lists, and throwing caution to the wind. I firmly believe that sex (and all it includes—emotional and physical connection) is one of the most important parts of a happy relationship. If you don't have that, your relationship will become less intimate in other ways, and then one day you'll wake up and realize you and your mate are living together more as roommates than lovers.

Once you have gotten back into the saddle and developed a routine that works for both of you, you can start to be a little bolder. Be spontaneous—greet him at the door wearing something sexy, his favorite drink in your hand, and a come-hither look on your face. Or, instead of jumping him at the door, take an opportunity to nurture him. Massage his feet and his back, make his favorite snack or drink, set up his favorite chair or side of the bed with some lotions and "toys" and play Florence Nightingale (nurse's costume optional). You see where I am going with this! Give date nights a try, but remember to be flexible. And, in addition to sex, focus on connecting with your mate during these special evenings; a simple dinner out (or a night in, if you're both wiped out) gives you time to just talk and listen, with no means to an end. Odds are these little exercises will lead to more and better sex.

It's really as simple as showing you're interested in and attracted to him. Doesn't everyone want someone to feel that way about them? Nothing is sexier than being desired, and having it reciprocated.

Try some of my tricks and come up with your own. Just put aside your fears, and get your mojo back! Your whole life will start to open up in ways that you've never imagined.

Marriage and Sex Quick Fix

I know, sometimes you just don't feel like "going there" in the bedroom. My advice is to just make yourself do it, and ninety-nine times out of one hundred you will be so happy you did. I guarantee that if you do, you will have a happy husband. (The female-focused version of the expression "happy wife, happy life" is "sexually satisfied husband, happy life"!) And besides, sex is great—it's fun and it feels good. So why not do it?

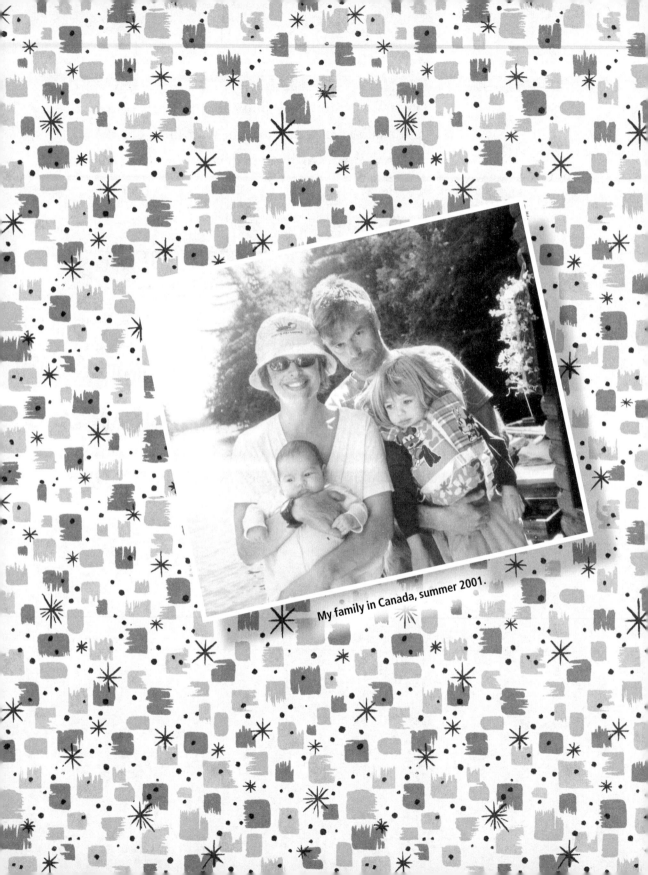

My family in Canada, summer 2001.

CHAPTER SIX

MOTHERHOOD MY WAY

If you bungle raising your children, I don't think whatever else you do matters very much.

—JACQUELINE KENNEDY ONASSIS

When my daughters were toddlers, I did all the modern mommy stuff. I took them to Mommy and Me classes, and a progressive preschool that taught children how to express themselves and mothers how to talk to them; I learned all the right and wrong things to do. But when Amelia was two, she went through a stage where she was spitting at people—at me, Harry, Delilah, anyone in her path. We tried to break her of this habit by using the techniques taught in the classes, but nothing seemed to be working. One day, we were in the kitchen, and she spit at me. Right then and there, all my "progressive" parenting lessons went out the window. I turned to her and said, "Listen, you do not spit. Girls do not spit, boys spit. If you don't stop spitting, you will grow a penis!" Delilah, who was five, looked at me in shock. Amelia never spit again. My response may not have been "by-the-book," but it worked! (I told my mother this story and she howled.) I am constantly improvising when it comes to parenting, and sometimes things like "don't do that or you will grow a penis" just fly out of my mouth. My girls think I am the kookiest mother around. I don't look or act like most mothers. I dance around the house, I'm clumsy, I don't cook, and I definitely have what I call my "I Love Lucy" moments.

I remember the day we brought Delilah home from the hospital. As we were strapping her into her infant car seat, Harry and I looked at each other, and both of our expressions said, *What do we do now?* Nobody gives you a handbook for parenting, and we were in uncharted territory.

Many of our friends had suggested we hire a baby nurse to show us the ropes and give me a break while I rested and recuperated. And, because no one tells you how to be a parent, you listen and do what your friends tell you to do. So we dutifully hired an English baby nurse, imagining it would be like having Mary Poppins in our home. (Although I doubt Mary Poppins arrived with the list of demands that this woman did. She presented us with a grocery list of specific foods, teas, and other beverages she required *for herself.* She also informed us that she must have her tea every day at 3 P.M. sharp. What did we know? We figured this was standard operating procedure.)

The very next morning after Mary Poppins's arrival, Harry walked into the nursery and found the nurse shaking Delilah and saying over and over, "Stop crying, no crying!" Harry left the room, called a cab, and the nurse was gone within the hour. So there we were, not even twenty-four hours after coming home from the hospital, completely on our own. In retrospect, it turned out to be a blessing in disguise, because it forced us to jump into parenthood feetfirst. Plus, my mother came and stayed with us for a few weeks, which was so comforting. She shared her wisdom and experience, and she got to watch her own daughter learn to be a mother, through trial and error.

However, there was one big elephant in the room, which I have never before talked about publicly: postpartum depression. Ten years ago, when I went through it, people just didn't talk about it. As a mother, I felt ashamed and filled with guilt. This was supposed to be the happiest moment of my life, and yet it felt like the worst. In recent years, many people have spoken out about it, including Brooke Shields and Marie Osmond, and some of the stigma has lifted, but I think it's still really hard for a mother to admit she's going through it.

I had severe postpartum depression with both my daughters. The first time, with Delilah, I had no idea what was happening to me. While I was pregnant, I felt the best I had ever felt in my life. I felt beautiful, sensual, and so blessed. After I gave birth, I descended into the darkest, scariest place, and was riddled with guilt. In fact, it was guilt times a thousand. I felt guilty about just being alive. Usually a mother suffering from postpartum depression feels guilty because she doesn't feel an immediate bond with her child, or is unable to experience the typical emotions of new motherhood. My experience was completely different. I felt hopeless and suicidal. I had horrific visions of knives, guns, and death. I would see myself stabbing Harry. I couldn't have any knives in the house. Harry had a gun, and I made him hide it where I couldn't find it. That's how real these visions were to me. I was afraid I might kill myself or my family. How scary is that?!

Since I didn't understand what was happening, I couldn't explain it to anyone else either. I tried talking to Harry and my mother, but I was so confused and ashamed that I couldn't articulate how bad it really was. They assumed I was just feeling tired and emotional, and that it would pass once I got a little rest.

Meanwhile, I knew how blessed I was to have a healthy baby girl, and a wonderful, supportive husband, but I couldn't control the visions in my head or get out of bed. The simplest task was overwhelming. I had no interest in my appearance. I lived in T-shirts and baggy sweats. Exercise had saved me every other time in my life, but this time it wasn't helping me. I tried to force myself to do it, but it didn't make me feel any better; nothing did. I was completely incapacitated.

I had been depressed before, and during those times I'd felt down on myself and negative. Postpartum depression is a totally different beast. (I call it a beast because it barges in and takes you over. I felt as if I were possessed. I swear, someone could have come in and done an exorcism on me.) You keep thinking it's going to get better tomorrow. That's why I didn't seek help from my doctor. Well, that and the shame I felt. My bout with postpartum depression went on for fifteen months! The thing that finally got me out of it was time and a job. I was offered a movie on the Lifetime channel called *Another Woman's Husband*, and my friend encouraged me to do it. I had to force myself to take it, but I did, and slowly I began to snap out of my depression. The cloud began to lift.

When I had Amelia three years later, I began experiencing the same postpartum symptoms I had suffered with Delilah. I felt hopeless, depressed, and unforgivably self-involved. When Amelia was about six weeks old, we were on the island in Canada we visit every August. I was trying to clean the cupboards, and I just couldn't do it. Instead, I sat on the kitchen floor and cried. I had to call my girlfriend and ask her to come help me. Harry recognized the signs of depression from after I had had Delilah, and convinced me to call my doctor in Los Angeles. Over the phone, he prescribed an antidepressant that he said would take about three weeks to kick in. During our phone call, my doctor explained postpartum depression to me this way: when you are pregnant, your hormones are sky-high, at approximately three thousand percent the usual levels. After you give birth, your hormone levels immediately plunge to zero. So if your body doesn't adjust automatically (as most women's hormone levels do), you have to reset them.

Once the antidepressants kicked in, the cloud totally lifted. They completely reset my hormonal clock. I finally cleaned those cabinets and the whole darned house! If only I had known to seek treatment after I'd had Delilah, I could have spared myself and Harry fifteen months of hell. I think it is so important for women to seek help if they think they might have postpartum depression. I don't care what anyone says, no amount of vitamins or exercise in the world could have helped what I was going through. The only thing that worked was the anti-depressant Serafem. I took them for about two and a half months, until I felt I didn't need them anymore, and I slowly went off of them under my doctor's supervision.

Every woman reacts to postpartum differently; it's a very individual thing. What was so strange about mine was I became the total opposite of who I am. I am usually going a million miles an hour, always active, very proactive, and optimistic. Though I wouldn't want to repeat those fifteen months, I don't regret them because the experience taught me a lot about myself and Harry. He was, as usual, my rock. Feeling so horrible about myself for so long made me appreciate how lucky I am to have the life and attitude (and husband) I do. Most importantly, it reaffirmed my belief in how important it is to both you and your family to feel good about yourself, no matter what it takes, because how you feel truly affects everyone and everything around you. As the old saying goes, "If Mama ain't happy, ain't nobody happy!" I had been a miserable mess.

As I mentioned earlier, it was absolutely wonderful to have my mother around when I was learning how to be a mom myself. My parents are extremely important forces in my life—I trace the person and mother I am today back to my parents and my own childhood, which was shadowed by tragedies suffered by both of my parents. When my mother was thirty years old, before she married my father, she was attacked and left for dead by a man who later became known as the "Trailside Serial Killer." Needless to say, this changed the way she approached life forever. After that experience, she was always cautious, overprotective, and afraid of taking risks. I grew up in an environment that was both loving and nurturing, but also surrounded by a lot of fear. But the most amazing thing about my mother is that she was able to overcome her own fears when it came to encouraging my dreams and goals. She was able to turn her fear around for my sake.

When it came to me, my mother never let her own feelings or apprehension get in the way of my aspirations, and I'm forever grateful for that. My mom is my hero, the woman I admire most in the world. She is the most forgiving woman I've ever known, and she always manages to turn a negative into a positive. That is an incredible gift to have and give to others, and one that I try to emulate every day of my life.

Both my parents were always very

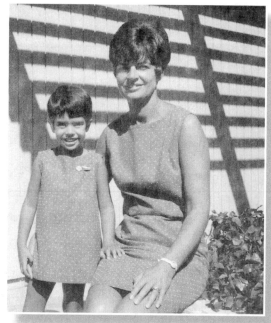

My mom and me, then three years old, wearing matching dresses.

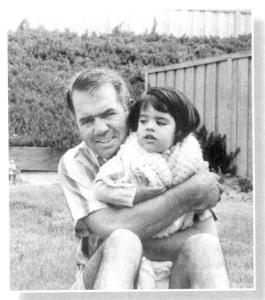
Dad and me when I was three, sharing a happy moment.

supportive of me and my dreams, but my mom in particular was never negative, or discouraging. She unfailingly believes that tomorrow will be a better day, and she always told me, "You can do it, you're great." Before her attack, my mom had dreamed of being an actress, so she took special joy in my success. When I got the part on *Days of Our Lives,* I was so excited because it had been one of my mother's favorite shows for years. We both thought it was the greatest thing in the world (so of course that is what it became!).

Like my mom, my father also suffered an unimaginable tragedy. When I was six years old, his then twenty-one-year-old daughter from his first marriage died from an accidental overdose of drugs and alcohol. As a young child, I didn't understand what had really happened. I just felt I had lost my father when his daughter passed away. Afterward, he was there physically, but emotionally something had changed. Now that I am a parent myself, I am better able to realize what he went through, and how horrific it must have been for him. (I cannot even conceive the pain of losing a child. That he managed as well as he did is a wonder and an inspiration to me.)

Both of my parents have endless sources of strength that never cease to amaze me. In a way, I became a natural survivor because of their experiences. It's a gift they gave me. I think I realized early on that life wasn't going to be easy and I needed to toughen up. As a child, I looked and acted different from the kids in Medford, so I was an easy target for my schoolmates, who called me names like "black cow" because I was dark-skinned (we didn't have a single black child in our school). They would also chant "The Diarrhea Song" at me (substituting "Lisa Rinna" for "diarrhea"), so that it became "Lisa Rinna, Lisa Rinna, people think it's funny, but it's really dark and runny." It was really hurtful. And I'll never forget an incident that happened when I was nine years old, around the age my daughters are now. I was walking across the playground during recess, and a boy threw a ball at my head so hard that it knocked me down. I was lying there on the ground, crying, with my underwear showing, and everyone was just watching me and laughing—no one even pretended to help me up. But I got back up, brushed myself off, and then and there resolved that they could knock me down but would never *keep* me down.

I instinctively knew that getting knocked down might just be my lot in life. I thank God that my daughters have not been subjected to that kind of teasing, but they have their own burdens to shoulder, and my childhood experiences help me to relate to whatever they may be going through. I can honestly tell them that I know exactly how they feel. When they are faced with bullying, I tell them to wish the bullies well, and send them a blessing; it's better to kill them with kindness than to fall prey to negativity. It doesn't always help my daughters feel better, but it's a good positive message. I admit I have told Delilah to stand up for herself by telling the bully, "That's not okay with me," and that if that doesn't work, give them a good sock in the face!

Another invaluable gift my parents, who have been together for forty-eight years, gave me is the example of a happy marriage. I think it is very hard to have a good relationship or marriage if you don't witness one firsthand. People tend to repeat what they know, whether it's good or bad. I saw that my parents genuinely liked each other; they were very compatible. They were also, like Harry and me, complete opposites. My father is artistic, a loner, and a thinker. My mom likes to be around people, to shop, and to stay busy (sound familiar?). She's a stickler for routine, and believes in everything in moderation, but most of all, she has the most positive attitude about life. My girls are lucky to see that they have a mother and father who love each other, and I hope they'll find the same kind of happy relationship themselves someday.

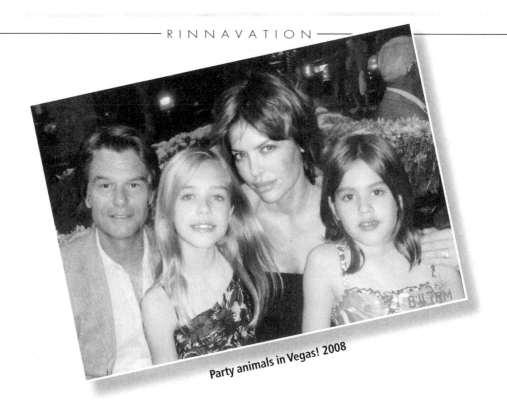

Party animals in Vegas! 2008

MOTHERHOOD MY WAY

My approach to motherhood is much like my approach to
life. I'm not perfect, I make mistakes, and I learn through
trial and error. None of us had a perfect childhood, but I
think we can learn from our parents' examples—both the
good and bad. I'm never going to be perfect. Just as my mom
did, I let my children know every day that I love them and
I hear them. They, in turn, know they can tell me anything,
and that with whatever they tell me, good or bad, I will stay
neutral. I try not to judge or jump in with advice. I just listen. More than anything, I think kids need to know they are
being heard, that what they say and do is important.

Answering the Tough Questions

As a parent, sometimes you get stumped. My feeling is, honesty is the best policy. Here's a recent example, so you can see this advice in action: my daughter Delilah and I were in the car, and she asked me if I had gone to college. *Okay, here goes*, I thought. *How do I answer this one? I'll just be straight with her.*

"I went to the University of Oregon for a term—"

"What's a term, Mom?"

"Well, it's about three or four months' worth of classes."

Then I continued to tell the story of why I dropped out, in a way that would teach her what I thought was a good lesson and would reinforce my values. I explained that I had wanted to be an actor so I signed up for Acting I (my very first acting class) in college. I loved it, and was excited to go on to Acting II. But you had to be accepted into Acting II—you couldn't just sign up—and my two Acting I teachers didn't put me into Acting II. I was devastated, and I quit. I told Delilah how hard the decision was and that I wanted to stay in school, but my passion was squelched for the moment. I also explained that I never gave up, that I found ways to make money while moving toward my goal, and that by refusing to let go of my dream I ended up where I am today. It was all about tenacity. I hope Delilah understood the messages I was trying to get across.

In addition to feeling loved and seen and heard, children must feel safe and protected. Childhood should be fun and free from worry and fear. It's about making them feel unconditionally loved and safe. This can be easier said than done, but it's a good goal, I believe.

Something else my parents taught me, that I try to instill in my daughters, is the importance of hugging and showing affection. My parents taught me not to be afraid to say *I love you.* This might sound obvious or simplistic, but I believe that all of us, at every age, need to constantly feel connected and treasured, to feel that we matter, and to feel confident enough to let other people know how we feel about them.

I try to teach my daughters the rules I live by, both through my words and actions. Stay true to who you are, don't try to be someone you aren't; and remember that everything that happens in our lives we create—we shouldn't blame others when something goes wrong. Instead, we have to ask ourselves, *What did I do to create this? How can I change it?* I don't think it's ever too early to teach this to our children. If my daughters are having trouble at school, whether with a classmate or a teacher, I ask them to think about what their part is in the situation. Often, once they think about it and take responsibility, they are able to see the situation and the solution more clearly.

I also have my family follow the "caught red-handed" rule. When one of us is caught in a lie or doing something wrong, we have to raise both hands in the air and say "caught red-handed." This is a way of taking responsibility for our mistakes, and it actually feels really good to do. My confession to Andrea Wong at the spinning class was a "caught red-handed" moment. And look at the good that came out of that! I tell my daughters stories like that to show them that I mess up all the time, but the important thing is to own up to it, which I do, and that owning up always lessens the impact of the mistake.

Another main component of my parenting philosophy is to encourage my girls to try new things and find their passions, and I support them if they discover something they enjoy. (But I make sure they know they don't have to be the best, or even have to stick with it, if it's not their thing.) For instance, Delilah takes horseback riding classes. It's not my favorite thing in the world to hang around stinky horse stalls all afternoon, but I do because I know she loves it. My mom did the same thing with me. If she hadn't encouraged my love of fashion by buying me magazine subscriptions, or indulging my passion for exercising by chauffeuring me to tennis lessons, I might not have discovered my true passions.

The No BS Rule
(This Rule's for the Parents!)

While I think it's incredibly important to encourage your kids to pursue their passions and follow their dreams, I also feel it's just as important to not bullshit them. If your child loves to sing and dreams of being the next Mariah Carey, but can't carry a tune in a bucket, you are not doing her a favor by telling her she is the greatest. Instead, help her focus on something she really is good at, and encourage that. Besides, kids have the best bullshit meters. They know when you are not being honest.

Don't get me wrong. I'm not saying you should only push your children to do something so they can be "the best" at it. In our society today, there is this disturbing concept that everyone has to be the best. Just go to any kids' softball game, and you will see it in action. It is usually the parents putting the pressure on. It's not about us, it's about them. Let them be kids, let them have fun, and yes, let them fail. Realizing that failure is not the end of the world is one of the most important lessons anyone can learn.

I love to push the boundaries, and this can be tricky to explain and pass along to my daughters, because obviously there's a good and a bad way to test the limits. But

I think they get that I like to put things out there so people will have a discussion about it, and that that discussion, hopefully, will lead to something positive. For instance, according to conventional wisdom, I shouldn't be posing in *Playboy*. But my hope is that I can be an inspiration to women by doing it. I am forty-five years old, a mother of two, and I have worked hard for this body, but people ask me how I am going to talk to my kids about the pictures. At this point, they are still too young for it even to register with them, but if it does, we will talk it through as a family. If it comes up, I will be honest with them. I want to show them it's okay to feel good about your body and yourself. I don't want them to feel secretive and shameful about their bodies and their sexuality. It's not something you can ignore and hope it will go away. This ties into my philosophy about the importance of feeling good about yourself. I see some mothers and it's obvious they have given up; they don't even try to look or feel good or try new things, and they've lost their identities. Many women resign themselves to "This is my life" or "I'm just dragging myself day to day." I think about the examples this sets for their children. Sure, we've all had our moment in the sun, and consciously or not, we want it back, but we just don't know how to do it. I say, figure it out now— it's never too late!

Balancing Work and Family

I think that by maintaining my drive and continuing to try to meet my personal and professional goals, I set another good example for my girls. I'm proud to be a working mom. So many women—I call us the "modern moms"—do this every day, and I know I am setting a good example for my daughters, just as my mom did with me. They see me juggling a million things, and hopefully they always know they are my number one priority. I want them to know that women can do anything and be career women, wives, and mothers all at the same time. I want to teach them compassion and kindness and giving, but I also want them to be strong women, to know that it's okay to ask for what you want, go after your dreams, stand up for yourself, and have a point of view. I want them to be able to say, "I don't like that, and that's not okay with me."

I go after my dreams, take risks, and am unafraid to be who I am; and I hope my daughters will be the same way. I have a lot on my plate, but I couldn't imagine living my life any other way. I never want my children to see me as a martyr, someone who gave up her dreams and life because of them. Not only does it put a heavy burden on children, it can also make you feel unfulfilled and resentful. Again, children learn by example. I think that if they see that you are happy and fulfilled, they grow up with the confidence and the tools to be happy and fulfilled themselves.

My secret to balancing my career and family is that when I'm doing something, I try to do it 100 percent; I am in the moment. When I am with the children, I am *with* them. They know it and they feel it. When I'm with the kids, I really pay attention—I try not to think about the grocery list or anything else. The same goes when I am working. Of course it's harder because, like most mothers, I am always thinking about the kids. If I am not with the family, my radar is up, but I think of it like meditating—

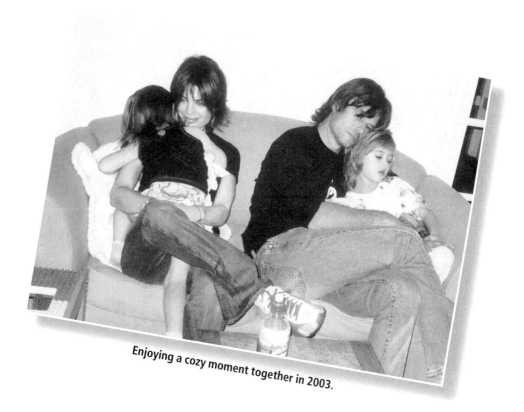

Enjoying a cozy moment together in 2003.

I just breathe and try to stay focused—and at the end of the day it makes me appreciate being with my family even more. And when I am with the kids and Harry, I don't have a care in the world. It's hard to do sometimes, but I believe it's the key.

You don't have to spend twenty-four hours a day with your kids, nor would they want you to. It's all about the quality of the time you do spend together. I think Harry is very good at spending quality time with our daughters. For example, the other day, the girls were playing hair

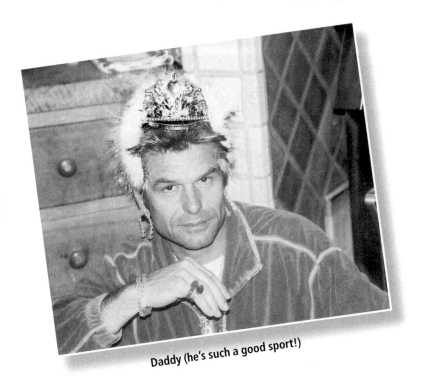

Daddy (he's such a good sport!)

salon, and Harry was the client. He had rubber bands in his hair. Can you picture that? He sat there for *hours* having his hair done. He is so patient. I, who am not so patient, learn from him every day. One of our sacred family traditions that ensures we spend quality time together is that Sunday is family day. We spend it together, just the four of us, and we try not to let anything interfere with that. No play dates, no exercise classes, nothing but us for the day. We make breakfast, go to the beach or to a movie, have lunch at a favorite restaurant . . . it's a special thing we all look forward to.

Mothering in the Spotlight

People often ask me how I think living in Hollywood with two parents in the public eye will affect my daughters. I don't really have an answer, but I know it's the only thing they have ever known, so they have no comparison. This is their reality, they don't know any different. Sometimes, my daughters' classmates will give them a hard time because they see them at a Jonas Brothers concert, or a movie premiere. It creates separation, and often envy. But I think they will turn out just fine, and it's my job to instill confidence, kindness, and a sense of groundedness in them to ensure that they do.

We recently had an interesting visit to Disneyland that served as a good learning experience. We had our own guide, and we didn't have to wait in line for the rides. Delilah previously had been to Disneyland with a friend, and she didn't receive any special treatment then, so she knew this was special, but Harry and I still made sure we explained that everything in life comes with benefits and sacrifices. While the girls appreciate the special perks, we try to make them appreciate the really important things in life—that they have a mom and dad who love each other and them. Fame and its trappings can disappear in a minute, but we will always have each other.

I just love the following passage from Marianne Williamson's *A Return to Love*, in which she interprets the Course in Miracles. It makes me think of my daughters, and I think if we can instill this message in our children, then we have given them the biggest gift.

"As I interpret the Course, 'your deepest fear is not that we are inadequate. Our deepest fear is that we are powerful beyond measure. It is our light, not our darkness, that most frightens us.' We ask ourselves, Who am I to be brilliant, gorgeous, talented, fabulous? Actually, who are you *not* to be? You are a child of God. Your playing small does not serve the world. There is nothing enlightened about shrinking so that other people won't feel insecure around you. We are all meant to shine, as children do."

Family Quick Fix

If you start to feel like your family seems disconnected, and you can't remember the last time you all did something together that wasn't a holiday or mandatory family reunion, plan a family date. Block off a couple of hours during the weekend and have a nice, long meal together, go for a hike, take a long drive through a beautiful area, do a project together like baking or putting photos into albums—anything that doesn't involve a television or work! That quality time is priceless.

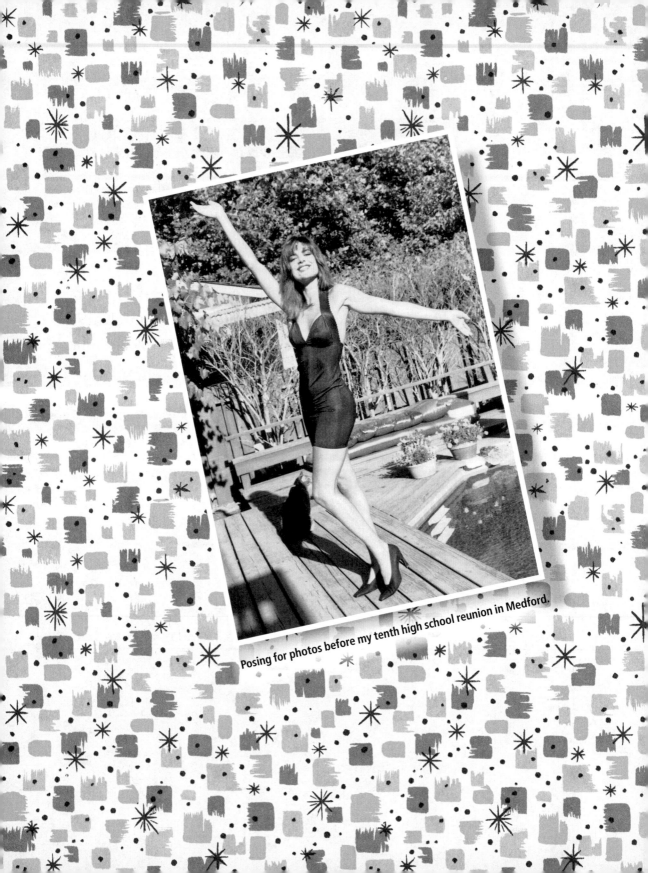

Posing for photos before my tenth high school reunion in Medford.

CHAPTER SEVEN

MY SPIRITUAL JOURNEY

*Life isn't about finding yourself. Life is
about creating yourself.*

—GEORGE BERNARD SHAW

Every summer, throughout my childhood, my family went to a resort in Oregon. We went with the same group of families at the same time every year, and it was always a great big reunion. One summer, when I was eight, I attached myself to a particular family, the Boilers. The Boilers had six kids, and were very devout Catholics. They went to mass every Sunday without fail. My mother and father weren't churchgoers, so I started tagging along with the Boiler clan. I loved everything about mass—the rituals and ceremony, the choir, and the feeling of being part of a group. Throughout my life, I've often felt like a loner and an outsider, never quite fitting in with my peers. I was an only child, after all, and so I loved the feeling of being welcomed and included. I think I was also searching for something to believe in, something bigger than me.

After attending mass with them a few times, I felt so comfortable with the Boilers, and so safe and accepted by the church, that one Sunday as everyone got up to take communion, I marched right up to the altar too. As I opened my mouth wide to receive the communion wafer, I felt all eyes on me. Everyone was looking at me in disbelief; the Boilers were temporarily mortified and the kids were nervously giggling. I had no clue that you couldn't just waltz up there and receive the body of Christ, that there was a whole process you had to go through first. But after that day, the Boilers anointed me an honorary Catholic, and I continued to attend mass with them for years. The story of my "first communion" became a running joke, but it really shows the strength of my convictions and beliefs, and the confidence they instilled in me even then.

In my teens, I was embraced by our neighbors, the Jones family. They were a large, rambunctious bunch and I adored hanging out at their house. As an only child, I loved feeling like part of a big family. Mrs. Jones was a dynamo, and way ahead of her time in many ways. She would take us to movies of all kinds, including some scary ones and intense dramas. I loved it! She was spontaneous and great fun to be around. Every Sunday, I accompanied the Jones family to their Presbyterian church for services. It was like mass with the Boilers all over again. I looked forward to it every week for the sense of purpose and belonging it instilled in me. One of the best parts was stopping at the local bakery for éclairs afterwards.

While I loved these experiences, I never did become a true convert to Christianity, never did communion and confirmation. As I would continue to do throughout my life, I took what I needed from each religion or spiritual practice and wove it into my life. I never totally devoted myself to any one practice, not from a lack of commitment, but instead an innate wariness of getting too swallowed up by any one idea or group. I always say that extremes don't work for me. I've seen people lose their identities that way—the group or the religion can become everything to someone, and suddenly there is no individual left. I like exploring new things, being open to many different things. My feeling is, why should I have to choose just one of anything when each has so much to offer?

I had been on a spiritual quest for years. I was always searching for the key that would unlock the door to true happiness, peace of mind, and well-being. Though I was generally outwardly happy, I always carried within me a feeling of unease, a sense that something was missing. Part of it is in the makeup of my personality. I'm always striving, searching; I never feel contented. I believe that the tragic events in my parents' lives subconsciously affected me. There is a line from the musical *Chicago* that says, "None of us got enough love in our childhoods. That's showbiz, kid." I think this is true for the majority of entertainers, who have a huge need for love and attention. It's certainly true for me. My parents were incredibly loving and supportive of me, and still are today. But they both lost pieces of themselves along the way, and subsequently they saw the world as a scary place. I must have picked up on this and internalized it. Maybe that is what led me to explore Christianity, and other spiritual practices.

In my twenties, I began devouring self-help books—*The Road Less Traveled, The Power of Positive Thinking, Feel the Fear and Do It Anyway*, and later *The Seat of the Soul.* (Basically, if it's been featured on *Oprah*, I've read it.) Though I first read some of these books almost twenty years ago, I often go back and re-read them, and every time I take something new from each one. I heard someone say that gleaning knowledge and making your way toward self-improvement is like planting seeds. They are not going to bloom overnight, but if you are patient and consistent, they eventually come to fruition. Sometimes it takes years and years. In my forties when I discovered *The Secret*, I finally found the key. That book completely changed my life. It opened the door for me to really understand for the first time that we create our own realities. I've always been quick to take action when I've felt that my life needed a change, but now I take a few steps first—I think, then feel, and *then* act, based on what I've learned over the past few years. And it wasn't that *The Secret* was saying anything profoundly different from all the other books I'd read. It was I who was different when I read it. I was ready.

The answers were there all along. But I had to have the experiences—the ups and downs—to be able to understand and appreciate them. I believe that every experience I've had, good and bad, has made me the person I am today. That is why I don't regret anything. For example, I know that the bad relationships in my past led me to Harry, because those relationships made me realize what I didn't want in a relationship and made me grateful for Harry and the relationship we developed and work to "perfect."

I was in therapy for eleven years during my twenties and thirties, much longer than I probably should have been. It's a good example of me thinking that I had more problems than I really did (a common occurrence in one's twenties and thirties). I started going at the urging of my then-boyfriend Peter. He was a big believer in therapy, and thought I would benefit. The therapist made me look deep into myself, which freed me to look at things I had been avoiding. I can't say it had a profound impact on my life, but then again, as often happens, maybe I just wasn't ready for it at the time. In any case, I eventually figured therapy wasn't helping—I wasn't happy, and I was still searching, so I stopped going. Much later, after Harry and I were married, I went to a very nurturing earth mother of a therapist for a few years. I felt so supported and grounded with her. When she died suddenly from cancer, I was devastated. I felt abandoned and adrift.

Harry and I went to a therapist together when we were about four years into our relationship. Basically, our problem was that he didn't want to get married and I did! We went for almost a year, we worked very hard, and a year later we got married.

Early on in our marriage Harry and I did phone sessions with a therapist who was a bit eccentric and unconventional (she was a thin, girl-like woman who was very intense and did therapy sessions out of a trailer behind her house!), but she gave us some valuable tools and helped us immensely. The most beneficial thing she taught us was to constantly ask ourselves if we needed each other. So many people confuse needing someone with being needy, but she showed us that asking the question and exploring the answer made the other feel valued, and important. Harry and I are both very independent, can-do people, and are loath to ask for help or admit we need something from the other. (This is one of the few things we have in common!) So now we make sure to let the other know that not only do we want each other, we also need each other. It sounds simple, but it's actually pretty complex and really powerful.

Harry and I also went to see a psychic who wore all white and lived in a white house. (I love a good psychic!) This was completely my idea. Harry is much more skeptical, while I tend to give anything a chance. She turned out to be more of a psychic/therapist; she was positive, supportive, and very insightful. I still check in with her every two years or so, whenever I feel stuck and need a jump-start. I view our sessions as digging into a toolbox: I take what I need at that time, whatever it takes to get my head into a good place, and then I go and try to fix whatever it is in my life that's bothering me. I feel very comfortable with and comforted by this woman. I saw her recently, and she told me I was very good at acclimating to life. At first, this seemed strange to me because I see myself as more proactive, a creator; and acclimating sounded so passive, like adapting or just accepting. She explained that she meant I was great at taking whatever was thrown at me and making it work. I guess it's a twist on the old "when life gives you lemons, make lemonade" maxim. I've had to do that a lot in my life!

About ten years ago, my friend told me about another amazing psychic. (If you suggest a psychic to me, I *will* go see her!) My friend had an actor-friend who had felt blocked in his career, and apparently this psychic had cleared out all the bad stuff that he was carrying around, and he got his career back on track in a big way. Her "office" was located in a little storefront next to the Trashy Lingerie store. When I walked in she looked at me and said, "You have so much bad stuff around you—it's like black soot, like someone put a curse on you." *Oy vey, now what?* I thought. "You always have felt people judging you, and you are putting out bad vibes." She then took an egg and dropped it in a basin of water. Then she took a sage stick, lighted it, and waved it around me. This is supposed to clear away all the bad karma. She had tons of oils for sale—for helping one find love, peace, harmony, you name it. I bought about twenty bottles! Because I had so much "black soot" (not to mention a bad spell) on me, she told me I had to go home and sit in a bath in freezing cold water, pour two quarts of goat's milk and white flowers over my head, and soak for twenty minutes in the frigid tub. You are now shaking your head, saying, "Lisa Rinna is crazy!" And I don't blame you. But what do you know, my life started to get better and better! Yes, maybe I am gullible. It could have been because I believed in it, and was open to potential effects, but whatever the reason, it worked for me.

I told Harry he had to see her. I guess he must have had even more black soot than I did, because she instructed him to do the white flower bath, but he had to sit in the freezing cold water for a full hour. The whole time he kept saying it was the dumbest, weirdest thing he'd ever heard of, and afterward, he got so sick that he almost got pneumonia. (Remember, Harry is the "smart one.") For the next five years, he kept getting cold after cold. To this day, he still gets colds all the time, and he blames that freezing bath. Obviously, it's not for everyone, but if you do try it, you have to be completely open and believe it. I think that a lot of what psychics offer—advice, predictions, home remedies—is self-fulfilling prophecy. If you think it's going to change your life for the better, it will. Thoughts are very powerful. They plant seeds, but you have to be open, to allow them to grow.

I went to see this same psychic recently for the first time in nine years, and she told me I was totally clean, I didn't have any of the black soot from before, and that I was right on track with my career and my business ventures. She then gave me two candles and three oils to help me work on my confidence and power. The candles were called The World at Your Feet and Success in Business. The oils were A Star Is Born, Horn of Plenty, and Wheel of Fortune. She instructed me to light the candles and not to blow them out but to let them burn all the way down. At the same time, I was to put drops of the oil into the candles and onto the bottoms of my feet. I also had to take two salt baths, one for confidence and one for power. Afterward, I felt great, fresh, and cleansed. And even though I knew that the candles, oils, and baths may not really have had any effect on my career, I think they helped keep me in a positive frame of mind.

Recently my friends told me about an East Coast–based psychic who was coming to Los Angeles. Of course I was first in line when he arrived. He told me I should live every day like it's a brand-new day. He said, "You have to stop thinking that your life has to be a struggle. You don't need to struggle; that is your idea. Just open yourself, treat every day like it's new, and start it with no preconceived notions. It doesn't have to be hard to be good." He also told me, "Your head is not connected to your heart. You need to write in your journal; you need to get your whole lifestyle message out there. You are very spiritual, and inspirational. You are a teacher." He didn't know I was writing a book, but his words made me think of the evolution of this book, which got so much deeper as I wrote it, connecting my head to my heart. I know all this talk about psychics sounds crazy, but I love a good visit with a psychic. It's fun, and the messages are always about staying positive and believing in myself and looking forward to the next thing, all of which I think are extremely important takeaways.

Around 2000, I became interested in Kabbalah. What I like about it is the belief that it is not what happens to us, it's how we react to it, or rather, how we don't. The idea is to be not reactive, but proactive. It's the difference between letting life happen to us or taking charge of what happens in our lives.

This speaks to me because it ties into my belief in taking responsibility for everything that happens, in being proactive, not passive or reactive. One thing I know for sure is that we create everything that happens in our lives, good and bad, and once we realize this, we can consciously start to create the lives we want. Kabbalah also urges people to treat others the way they want to be treated, and reinforces the importance of giving and helping others—lessons that are covered in many religions and that I try to remember as often as I can. Another tenet of Kabbalah that appeals to me is the belief in free will. Unlike some practices, it doesn't say that your life is predestined and that you have no control over what happens. If that is the case, then where's the motivation to make things happen?

I believe you can choose the way you think, and what kind of energy you put out there—that like attracts like. If you believe that good things will happen, they will. As simplistic as this may sound, think about the kind of people you like to be around, the kind of life you want to have. You will only attract these things if you are like-minded. You might not get what you're wishing for right when you want it, but you will get it when you are ready for it. We can only achieve this if we stay open and engaged, and believe. It's all about putting it out to the universe. As *The Secret* says, "Ask, believe, receive." My main philosophy is, *What do I have to lose?* Look what I stand to gain!

Most people, myself included, often think happiness is what you feel when you get the big job, or the dream house, or the fancy car, or the pined-after lover. But we want the feeling, the joy or exhilaration that getting something brings, not the thing itself. The satisfaction of getting it is what we are all really searching for, not the material item itself, but the emotion we experience when we achieve that goal or get that car. I know this may sound funny coming from an avid shopper like me, but I try to balance the material, or outer, things with the spiritual, or inner, things.

I try to force myself to think about the feelings and emotions I get when I have acquired or accomplished something big. It might be self-satisfaction, pride, triumph, joy, exhilaration, gratitude, or euphoria. Then my goal is to get this feeling from my life, and from the people in my life, not things. It's about quality, not quantity. I believe that if we feel good about ourselves, our bodies, our lives, if we love who we are and accept ourselves for who we are, that's when life is sublime. That to me is true happiness.

I also try to think about what I want my legacy to be. At the end of my life, what do I want to be remembered for? What do I want to have accomplished? In one of the acting classes I took in my twenties, we did an exercise called "superlatives," in which each of us had to choose a character or action and be the very best at it, whether that meant the best clown or drunk or cheerleader, you name it. The lesson was to be the very best you can be in anything you do. Along the way in life, as you change and grow, I think the definition of your "very best" changes, but as long as it's *your* very best, you will stay on the right path. This goes hand in hand with staying true to yourself and not trying to be anything you're not.

Another element that is key to my spiritual well-being is gratitude. I believe that once you learn to truly appreciate all of life's gifts, you begin to receive more and more. Louise L. Hay, the legendary self-help author and teacher, says, "The universe really loves gratitude. And the more gratitude you have, the more goodies you get." One big lesson I've learned about gratitude is that it starts with me. I have to be grateful for my life as it is right now, to myself, for the person I am, for what I've survived, for the person I want to become. I try to thank myself for everything I do, every day. This is incredibly hard for most people, myself included, to do. But if you feel good about yourself, if you realize your worth and your contribution to the world, everyone benefits. You'll attract good things, and others will benefit from your positivity; the same things happen if you feel bad—you'll put negative vibes out into the world, and attract more of the same.

THE POWER OF A POSITIVE ATTITUDE

People are afraid to pursue their most important dreams, because they feel that they don't deserve them, or that they'll be unable to achieve them.

—PAULO COELHO

Eight years before I did *Dancing with the Stars*, I auditioned for the role of Velma in *Chicago* on Broadway, which was a harder dance role than the Roxy role. I had no formal dance training at that point, and I looked like the biggest fool onstage trying to keep up with the moves. Needless to say, I didn't get the part.

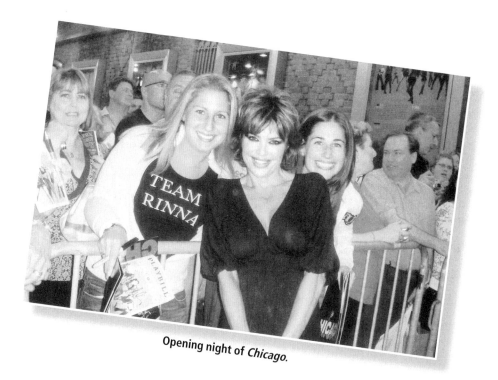

Opening night of *Chicago.*

After *Dancing with the Stars*, I went into my agent's office with a list of things I wanted to accomplish. To date, I'm proud and surprised to say, I've accomplished every single thing on that list. And yes, one of the items was starring in *Chicago* on Broadway. Three months after *DWTS* ended, my agent approached the *Chicago* producers, who have long memories, and they weren't all that interested. So, on my own dime, I flew myself to New York and put myself up at a hotel. I hired a singing coach, who worked with me on the songs. I also worked with Greg Butler, the *Chicago* dance captain in New York. I worked really hard and prepared three songs and a monologue. For the audition, I wore a little short skirt and fishnet stockings (products from my *DWTS* days) and danced and sang my heart out. It was a totally humbling experience—after all, they had rejected me outright once and had basically rejected me indirectly a second time. But I did well, and I never would have gotten the part if I hadn't taken a big risk and worked really hard. It was as scary and difficult as it was ultimately rewarding.

If I want something really badly, I put as much positive energy toward achieving my goal as humanly possible. Take soap operas—everyone looked down on them back when I was trying to land acting jobs. I took my role on *Days of Our Lives* and made it into something great, because I thought what I was doing was the coolest thing ever. In my house, when I was growing up, soap operas were cool. My mom had watched *Days of Our Lives* for years; so for me, landing a role on the show was one of the greatest coups of my career. Had I gone into it thinking it was beneath me, that it would make me look like a loser, that's what would have happened. Working hard and believing in myself and what I'm doing has brought me the success I've been lucky to have.

I try to look at everything as an opportunity. I've found that usually the things we least want to do are the things that reap the biggest benefits. So many times I don't feel like going to a meeting or party, but then I try to think of what good might come out of it. I might meet a life-long friend, or run into someone I haven't seen in years. Many times, attending an event has resulted in invaluable professional connections, so I push myself. I am all about evolving, finding the next thing. I try not to fixate or obsess on things. I just take what I want from them, and move on to the next one.

I haven't always been able to block out the negatives and keep facing forward. It's taken a lot of work and discipline to develop my current attitude. I've had some very dark periods in my life, especially when I wasn't working. I would constantly compare myself to my more successful friends during these times, and my envy took a toll on me. I was jealous of other people's houses, careers, and relationships. I had been acquainted with envy since I was a child. As much as I loved the Jones family, I was jealous of their big, boisterous lives. I always felt that I didn't have enough, that I wasn't enough. The same tape kept playing over and over.

I think my turning point was participating in *Dancing with the Stars*. That experience put me in a positive place that I'll always strive to maintain. I felt so great, and all these good things started to come along, and I thought, *I want this all the time*! Then I read *The Secret*—and suddenly it all made sense to me. Previously, I had been putting out a lot of negative energy, and that's what I had been getting back. If I feel negative or depressed, I make sure I do something to change it, so that I don't attract more negativity and bad things into my life. I'll smile at everyone I see. I'll ask the clerk at the grocery store how her day is going. It forms a chain reaction. I also realized that there is enough positive energy to go around, and that we should never compare ourselves to other people.

When Partying Pays Off

In December of 2007, I attended a Christmas party that I wasn't exactly in the mood to attend. While there, I met a photographer named Deborah Anderson. She was in the middle of shooting a coffee table book for charity called *Room 23* that depicted what may have taken place in a specific hotel room over the course of a year. Deborah showed me some of the photos she'd taken on her iPhone, and they were amazing. She'd already taken photos of Cindy Crawford, George Clooney, Elton John, Sharon Stone, and Lindsay Lohan, and she asked if I would pose for the book too. I was beyond flattered. I said yes, but I told her that I wanted to pose nude. (Yes, I just blurted that out. How weird is that?)

I just knew she would find a way to make the photos gorgeous and sophisticated and classy. It was my gut feeling again.

We did the shoot, during which I posed both naked and wearing sexy lingerie. It was fantastic; I felt so free the entire time. After I saw the pictures, I said to Deborah, "We should do this for *Playboy*." It turns out that Deborah was in talks with the people at *Playboy* and was really eager to shoot for them, so I told her to send some of the photos from our shoot to the magazine, and we'd see what they said.

Now I knew Harry wouldn't be crazy about the idea. Ten years earlier I had appeared on the cover of *Playboy* while I was seven months pregnant with Delilah, and I was certain he would say, "No way, you already did it!" if I brought up the fact that I wanted to pose for them again. So when I got home, I showed him the shots, but I waited until we heard back from *Playboy* to disclose my "plan." They called about a month later and said, "Let's do it," and it was time to convince Harry!

I went into our bedroom, gave him my best "This is why I should do *Playboy*" speech, and, as I predicted, he was against it. But Harry saw I had that look in my eye that I get when I want something really badly and I've already made up my mind. And he eventually said, "Go for it." I wouldn't have done it if he had really stuck to his guns and remained against it; it had to be a joint decision. Harry actually ended up thinking it was the greatest thing—the photos are so classy and artistic, we were thrilled with the outcome.

Thankfully, even in my darkest times, I never turned to drugs or alcohol, or had any eating disorders. I guess I knew instinctively that I needed to feel things, and stay healthy in order to come through the experience. My motto has always been, *Everything in moderation.* I inherited this from my mother and my father, who are very moderate in everything they do. I've never seen either of them drink too much; my mother never even overate. I admit to control issues about my weight, and I am always conscious of it (this is not so unusual for an actress, but I know I would feel the same even if I weren't in this business), but I don't fall victim to extremes, and my respect for my body keeps me in check.

I realize I am very fortunate that I've never had an addictive personality. I think there is a fine line between passion and addiction. I consider something a passion if I enjoy it *and* can weave it successfully into my life, in a way that enhances my life. If it's an addiction, it is not going to benefit me or my life in any way, so I leave it alone.

Over the years, my true passions in life haven't changed, but the way I look at them has. I used to play down my passions—fashion, exercise, and the entertainment world. I feared seeming shallow and superficial. I felt I should be more serious, more educated. What changed is I learned to accept myself, and appreciate my passions as talents. That changed everything, and gave me the motivation to build my businesses. Accepting myself has been the hardest and most rewarding step I've ever taken. My appearances as a guest host on *Regis and Kathie Lee* (before they hired Kelly Ripa as Regis's permanent cohost) caught the attention of the people who did *Soaptalk* because I was just being myself. Later, when I was hosting *Soaptalk* in 2000, I was working without a script and had to rely on my wits. My true self really came out—I am clumsy, I'm a goofball, and I can't cook. Instead of beating myself up or making excuses, I made fun of myself, and it became a running gag on the show. It gave me confidence because I was being true to myself, and it was working. That experience, in turn, really prepared me for my current red-carpet gig for the TV Guide Network, where I engage people by being myself—after all, there's no room for posturing as a red-carpet reporter.

While being comfortable with myself has helped me come a long way, I also think it is so important to have role models, people you admire, respect, and look up to.

My role models are women who excel at being mothers, wives, businesswomen, or just a really good girlfriend. I am a big fan of Cindy Crawford, Demi Moore, Madonna, and Goldie Hawn, because they work very hard to constantly be their best at all they do. They are great mothers, have strong relationships, and have built long careers. They are very spiritual and are constantly evolving and growing.

I also really admire people who do what they want and don't judge others or worry about what other people think. I'm all about making personal choices, and I don't think you should be judgmental and negative about others who don't agree with you. You should do whatever you need to do to feel good about yourself. I've seen women with gray hair and no makeup who look stunning. I also know firsthand how a little hair color or lipstick can make a big impact in terms of improving your attitude. I want to stay fresh and at the top of my game, take risks, try new things, even if they don't always work out the way I wanted. I want to look good for my husband and for myself. I believe that you have to keep growing up, searching for new answers, being open to new opportunities, and all the while be grateful for every day and every experience.

Motivational Quick Fix: Take a Personal Inventory

It is never too late to be who you might have been.

—GEORGE ELIOT

Every so often I stop and take stock of my life. I ask myself:

- Where was I five, ten, twenty years ago?
- How have I changed over the years?
- What did I imagine my life would be like now?
- Where would I like it to be five years from now? What about ten years from now?
- What is the thing I fear the most but would give my right arm to do?

Get a pad of paper and take stock of your life. Ask yourself these questions or make up your own. Really let your mind go and dream big. Be specific, right down to where you are, what you are wearing, who is there with you, and how you feel. I believe everyone can and should have a dream and identify and experience their big moment. It's never too late.

CONCLUSION

After I hosted the Screen Actors Guild awards in January of 2008 for the TV Guide Network, the legendary Howard Stern, whom I barely know, called me out of the blue and generously offered me some constructive criticism. On air he critiqued the way I was dressed (of course, he wanted to see more skin), told me to take my lips down (which I did), and told me I had to listen more. He also said I had to ditch my "fake laugh." I didn't get defensive, I really listened—that surprised me! Prior to the SAG awards show, I had only done the Emmys show in September of 2007 (where I felt very comfortable because of my television background). Howard is so smart—it would be idiotic *not* to listen to him. I figured I could only get better, and it felt really good to be able to admit that.

I hosted the Grammy awards not long after our phone call, and the following week I appeared on Howard's show. On the air, he talked about our phone call and commended me for following his advice and told me how much better

I had done. (Of course, he also told me I still had a lot of room for improvement!) Though I had done a few phone interviews for his show in the past, I had never been face-to-face with him in the studio before. In my thirties, when I was acting on *Melrose Place*, I was invited to do the show and said, "No way, I can't handle it." I didn't have the confidence. After *Dancing with the Stars*, nothing seems to scare me much anymore. I just tried to be myself, to be as real as possible. I think that the older you get, and the more comfortable in your body you are, the more real you become, and you stop caring so much about what people think. In my twenties (and thirties), I never would have been able to handle Howard Stern. But now I thought I could. Not only that, I ended up having a blast on his show!

When I hosted the Oscars awards show later that month, it didn't go well at all. It was my toughest show yet. The Golden Globes awards show in January had been canceled due to the writers' strike. I had really been looking forward to the Golden Globes because it's similar to the Emmys but more relaxed and fun. Plus I needed the practice. After the Oscars show, I was down on myself. I felt nervous and insecure. The following week, I was called to a meeting with the TV Guide Network executives. They sat me down and showed me clips from the shows I had done. First they showed me the ones they thought were great, and then they showed me the ones they thought didn't work. And those didn't stop. After they showed me about five of the bad ones, I thought, *Okay, I get it!* But then they showed me another and another. We were in this huge conference room, and I was watching myself on an equally enormous plasma screen, trying to stay open to what they were saying, while trying not to cry. My agent, Jonathan, was sitting beside me, and he was as blindsided as I was. Neither of us had expected this. (Though I don't think it would've been any less brutal if we had known.)

In retrospect, I realized they were just trying to help me. They thought that Howard Stern had freaked me out when he pointed out all the things I needed to improve on, and that had made me self-conscious. Maybe Howard had a little bit to do with it, but my rocky performance was the result of a variety of things. It was a huge learning curve, and I had to figure it out for myself. Not only did I have to learn the ropes and weather the inevitable criticism, but I also had to deal with the rejection—there were certain celebs who wouldn't talk to me. Their handlers decide whom they should talk to. I knew I shouldn't take it personally; it was just part of playing the game. Still, it took a toll on me.

As an actress, I'm used to reciting lines written for me, and a director telling me what to do. When I am live on the red carpet, there is no one giving me direction or feeding me lines. I've had to learn to go with the flow and stay on my toes, instead of thinking about the next question I'm going to ask. Luckily for me, I discovered that I do my best when I just allow things to happen—*whatever happens happens.* What the execs loved the most were the spontaneous moments, when I would mess up or something would come out of my mouth that you would never expect. I think we all want to see people being real. The viewers want to see the chemistry and the relationship (or sometimes the lack thereof!) between me and the celebrity I'm interviewing.

Despite the best intentions of the TV Guide people, sitting there in that conference room was one of the most difficult things I've ever had to do. But I did sit there, and I listened and said, "You're right. I hear you." They didn't want me to explain or make excuses. They wanted me to listen. It's devastating when you've worked really hard and someone says, "I don't like the way you did that" (whether it's a meal you've slaved over or a project at work you've put your all into). But I try to look at everything as a learning experience (not always successfully, I might add). It's up to me how I respond. I can get angry and resist, or I can turn it into something positive. I've also had to work on developing a tough skin while staying open at the same time.

The whole red-carpet experience made me realize how far I've come over the years, particularly in how I react to things. I don't take things so personally, I don't get defensive or angry (well, not as much!), and I strive to keep learning and growing, in every area of my life. In other words, I try to walk the walk and talk the talk. It also made me think about the evolution of this book. As I mentioned in the introduction, this book originally started out as a beauty, fitness, and fashion book. But as I began looking back over my life, I started to see certain patterns. I realized how much I had changed (for the better, hopefully!), and how everything that happened to me happened for a reason. It wasn't always obvious at the time, but I was on my own personal journey, and it was up to me to direct it, to create my own story. I took my passions and figured out a way to use them to create the life I wanted. So many things in my life that might have seemed accidental at the time—meeting Harry, doing *Dancing with the Stars*, hosting for the TV Guide Network— could easily have gone nowhere if I hadn't grabbed them with both hands, and worked like the devil to turn them into something fabulous.

I know I look and feel better today than at any other time in my life because of (not in spite of!) all I've been through. Harry says I've grown into my features and I'm more beautiful now than when we met (I think that's a compliment!). That's one of the reasons I decided to pose for *Playboy* magazine again. Ten years earlier, in 1998, I appeared on the cover when I was six months pregnant with Delilah. Both times, it was my idea, and I approached the magazine. At forty-five, I feel more comfortable in my body and my sexuality than at any other point in my life. I think it's something to celebrate, and it's a good message for all women who feel that life, or their sexuality, ends at forty, or after childbirth. That is why I deliberately chose a photographer who would make the pictures classy and sexy at the same time.

WHERE I AM TODAY

All my life I've never thought I was beautiful, so it's ironic that I ended up in a business and live in a culture that puts so much emphasis on beauty. I have worked hard to make myself feel beautiful, but the truth is, I still feel like that little seven-year-old girl with the dark skin, short dresses, and odd features. Maybe the unease I have felt in my life is just a part of growing up—maybe we all feel this way and that is what makes us search for more. But it is also what has made me who I am today. What I have discovered is that *there is no key; there are no shortcuts.* It sounds clichéd, but it really is all about the journey—your journey, my journey. We all have one.

One of my goals in writing this book was to share some of my journey with you. My hope is that it will help you in some way, shape, or form. I don't claim to be an expert on much of anything, but what I do know is that how you think and feel creates your life. You really can change your story at any time in your life. I used to think it was all about taking action to change your life, but I am now learning it is about having the thought first, the feeling second, and then the action third. Though it sounds complex, it's actually easier in a way because you can take baby steps—first you think about it, then you experience the feelings it evokes, and finally, if it feels right, you take action. So why not—starting right now—get the life that you want, no more excuses? Take what you have and make a masterpiece!

If you feel bad about yourself, do something, anything, to change that feeling! Get up and do something, set a goal for yourself. Get the (you fill in the blank) of your dreams. Be abundant and grateful in love, money, and good health. Help a friend, or give your time or money to a hospital or

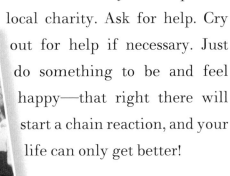

local charity. Ask for help. Cry out for help if necessary. Just do something to be and feel happy—that right there will start a chain reaction, and your life can only get better!

ACKNOWLEDGMENTS

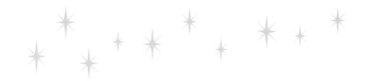

Mom and Dad, I love you. Thank you for your support and guidance.

Fred, I'd be lost without you, baby! You are my rock.

Jonathan, thank you, you are a guardian angel. Can you believe we finally did it? Next on the list is . . .

Bill, thank you for always being there. I couldn't do it without you.

Fritzo, you are one of a kind, and I thank God for you!

Prophet, you rock!

Faye, luv you!

Adam, come on now!

Bruce, my happy companion and friend, you help me every day.

Lyndie, my soul sista—without you I am nothing.

Jana and Robin, you have my back and I'll never forget that.

Heather and the girls at Belle Gray, thanks for putting up with my craziness. You are all the best!

Guerin, you are always there for me, and I so appreciate it.

Jen Rade, thanks for making me look fab!

Nancy, Dorrie, and Traci, thanks for always being supportive.

Ninie, without your help nothing would get done. Thank you!

Deena, thank you for all of your support and love.

Maureen O'Neal, what a journey. Thanks for taking it with me!

Mrs. Claus, thanks for the inspiration, always.

Emily Westlake, thank you for taking this project under your wing and making me feel protected.

Jen Bergstrom, thanks for believing in me and my book, and for believing that I had a story to tell.

Dan Strone, thanks for believing in this project too.

Kate Somerville, thanks for all the great facials and changing my skin!

Dr. Lancer, thanks for helping me be zit free and getting rid of the spots.

Jeff, thanks for everything—my body is nothing without you!

Louie V., you have been there for three years, and you

changed my life! Thank you so much for all that you have done and your patience in teaching me how to dance.

Sheila Kelley, thanks for the gift of the S Factor. It changed my life!

Lou Paget, you also changed my sex life forever. Thank you, and my husband thanks you!

June, wherever you are, thank you!

Kevin K., you have always been such a good friend.

Lorena, thank you for all that you do for us!

Howard Stern, thank you for your encouragement and support.

To everyone at the TV Guide Network, thanks for giving me the job of my dreams!

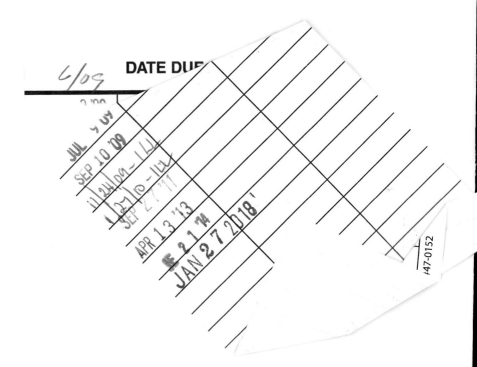

DATE DUE

6/09

JUL

SEP 10 '09

SEP 27 '11

APR 13 '13

JAN 27 2018

47-0152